Nursing and Collaborative Practice

A Guide to Interprofessional and Interpersonal Working

Transforming Nursing Practice series

Transforming Nursing Practice links theory with practice, in the context of the skills and knowledge needed by student nurses to be fit for future healthcare delivery. Each book has been designed to help students meet the requirements of the NMC Standards for Pre-Registration Nursing Education, Essential Skills Clusters and other relevant competencies. They are accessible and challenging, and provide regular opportunities for active and reflective learning. Each book will ensure that students learn the central importance of thinking critically about nursing.

Series editor:
Dr Shirley Bach, Head of the School of Nursing and Midwifery at the University of Brighton.

Titles in the series:

To order, contact our distributor: BEBC Distribution, Albion Close, Parkstone, Poole, BH12 3LL. Telephone: 0845 230 9000, email: **learningmatters@bebc.co.uk**. You can also find more information on each of these titles and our other learning resources at **www.learningmatters.co.uk**. Many of these titles are also available in various ebook formats. Please visit the website above for more information.

Nursing and Collaborative Practice

A Guide to Interprofessional
and Interpersonal Working

Second Edition

Benny Goodman and Ruth Clemow

LearningMatters

BP45

First published in 2008 by Learning Matters Ltd
This edition published 2010

British Library Cataloguing in Publication Data
A CIP record for this book is available from the British Library

ISBN: 978 1 84445 373 3

This book is also available in the following ebook formats:

Adobe ebook   ISBN: 978 1 84445 677 2
EPUB ebook   ISBN: 978 1 84445 676 5
Kindle   ISBN: 978 1 84445 979 7

Cover design by Toucan Design
Text design by Code 5 Associates Ltd
Project Management by Diana Chambers
Typeset by Kelly Winter
Printed and bound in Great Britain by TJ International Ltd, Padstow, Cornwall

Learning Matters Ltd
33 Southernhay East
Exeter EX1 1NX
Tel: 01392 215560
E-mail: info@learningmatters.co.uk
www.learningmatters.co.uk

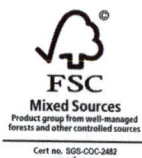

FSC
Mixed Sources
Product group from well-managed
forests and other controlled sources
Cert no. SGS-COC-2482
www.fsc.org
© 1996 Forest Stewardship Council

6/13/11

Contents

Foreword

Nursing is a far from solitary occupation. We constantly interact with colleagues, patients and peers in the working environment. As human beings we should be well equipped to do this with our natural instincts and the social learning opportunities we have had in life. However, there are many examples of investigations and reports into health and social care situations that have gone disastrously wrong because of poor collaboration and communication between fellow workers. In this text, Goodman and Clemow have revised the first edition and provide an up-to-date tool box of ideas and explanations for improving the quality of how we work together and collaborate with others.

As well as an interesting read, it should be an essential text on the nursing curriculum to assist students in learning the whys and wherefores of how working together can be better understood and more effective. The text takes time to explore many terms and definitions of language that have emerged from history, policies and organisational 'speak', with activities and examples to illustrate. Words do not always mean the same thing to individuals and misunderstandings of meanings can lead to ineffective working together – which is why time spent in this text on explanations is so crucial.

There is also a lively and critical edge to the text which brings to the surface, by asking questions and reflecting, some of the issues we face when working with colleagues; such as our responses to different cultural mores and perspectives on the doctor–nurse relationship and sterotyping. It also provides guidance on working in different settings such as rural, mental health and child health.

There are practical and theoretical examples to delve deeper into the workings of teams, drawing on social psychology theory. Lecturers and students will find the text helpful in understanding the merits and disadvantages of interprofessional education and learning.

In sum, you will enjoy this text as it deals with everyday working, providing a valuable guide to working with others effectively. In each chapter the relevant NMC *Standards for Pre-registration Nursing Education* and NMC Essential Skills Clusters are stated and will be a feature of the Transforming Nursing Practice series. This ensures nursing students will see exactly how the information in the book relates to achieving their competencies and be ready to practise in the contemporary world of nursing we know today.

Shirley Bach
Series Editor

Acknowledgements

The authors and publishers would like to thank the following reviewers of the first edition for their helpful suggestions for improvements to the second edition:

Lynne Westwood, University of Wolverhampton
Paul Elliott, Canterbury Christ Church University
David Gallimore, Swansea University
Keith Booles, Staffordshire University
Caroline Sargisson, Middlesex University
Alan Pringle, University of Nottingham
Kim Hanson, University of Cumbria

Introduction

Who is this book for?

This book is primarily for students of nursing. The focus is not to develop knowledge for any one specific branch (Adult, Child, Mental Health or Learning Disabilities) but to support development for *any* branch and beyond. Therefore, there may well be value for those who are studying on branch programmes and those on continuing professional development modules. It may also be of interest to experienced nurses who have mentoring roles. The Nursing and Midwifery Council's draft *Standards for Pre-registration Nursing Education* are a foundation for what follows. However, the content is not narrowly defined by them.

Working with other people – interprofessional and interpersonal practice

Working with other people is a fact of everyday life. Whether you will be working as a practitioner in primary care with your own case load, or whether you will be embedded within an operating theatre team in an acute hospital, you will be constantly interacting with other people in order to assess, plan, implement and evaluate your care. You will also experience the various changes to care delivery that come from government and employers' policies. The pace of change in the provision of health services in all likelihood will not slow down. The previous changes have meant examining how the various professions have had to rethink and reconfigure what they do.

Nursing work is thus largely 'people work', whether it is the one-to-one patient encounter or providing team-based care.

A note on terminology

The use of 'patient/client/service user' is not to assume that we always mean hospital in-patients. We will often refer to 'people', but when the context demands we will use 'patient' or 'client'.

Draft Standards for Pre-registration Nursing Education

These standards (NMC, 2010) are used by those planning courses for nursing education. At the beginning of each chapter will be a guide to the most pertinent domains and competencies described in the standards. The NMC has also published draft Essential Skills Clusters with the standards. Therefore, we will identify some of the 'essential skills' that need to be achieved throughout the educational programme. Again, at the beginning of each chapter we will highlight those skills to which the chapter may contribute. However, this may not be exhaustive and users should consult the full standards to support their own learning. The four domains, with their respective generic standards for competence, are as follows.

1. Domain: Professional values

- Graduate nurses must act to safeguard the public, making people their first concern. They must be responsible and accountable for safe, compassionate, person-centred, evidence-based nursing care and interventions. They must show professionalism, integrity and caring, working, in partnership with people and their carers and other health and social care professionals and agencies, within professional, ethical and legal frameworks.

2. Domain: Communication and interpersonal skills

- Graduate nurses must have 'presence' demonstrated through the energy and quality of their interaction. They must communicate safely and effectively with individuals and groups of all ages, using a variety of complex skills and interventions including communication technologies. Communication must be characterised at all times by respect for individual differences, care, compassion and dignity.

3. Domain: Nursing practice and decision making

- Graduate nurses must practise in a compassionate, respectful way, maintaining the dignity and wellbeing of all concerned. Decision making must be person-focused, and through a process of critical analysis leading to a range of technical skills and nursing interventions from basic to highly complex. They must practise in a safe and confident manner, in various care settings, understanding how the environment and location of care delivery can have an impact on health and outcomes. All practice must be based on current evidence and up-to-date technology.
- Nurses must demonstrate a knowledge and understanding of how lifestyle, diversity and socio-economic factors can affect health and illness and public health priorities. They must meet the needs of people of all ages who may have overlapping physical and mental health problems, such as: children and young people with addiction problems, eating disorders, learning disabilities; adults with depression, eating disorders, dementia, drug and alcohol abuse; older people with dementia, restricted life styles due to disability, long term illness.

4. Domain: Leadership, management and team working

- Graduate nurses must be professionally accountable and use clinical governance processes to maintain and improve standards of health care and nursing practice. They must be able to respond autonomously and confidently to planned and uncertain situations, managing themselves and others effectively, creating and maximising opportunities to improve services. They must also demonstrate the potential to develop further management and leadership skills during their preceptorship and beyond.

Links to the pre-2010 standards relevant to this book are outlined on the Learning Matters website page for this book **www.learningmatters.co.uk/nursing**. Updates with the final standards will also be available on this website.

NMC Essential Skills Clusters

The NMC states that the Essential Skills Clusters (ESCs) must be put into all pre-registration nursing programmes. How this is done is left to those who are planning the educational experience. There are five skills clusters in total:

- care, compassion and communication;
- organisational aspects of care;
- infection prevention and control;
- nutrition and fluid management;
- medicines management.

These ESCs are designed to support the achievement of the competencies listed under each of the four domains. Some chapters in this book are particularly relevant to certain clusters, and this will be highlighted as appropriate.

Book structure

The title of the book points you to consider that nursing is about working collaboratively. However, it is also about interpersonal work, meaning that nursing work is people work . . . you are 'working with other people'.

In Chapter 1, 'Working with other people', we will explore what is meant by working with other people. We will examine the many terms and phrases used in the health literature and by the professional groups. We need to understand the term 'people' to emphasise that it is not just about working in teams with other professionals; it is also about the patient, client and service user.

In Chapter 2, 'The context: history and policy', we will discuss the history of, and policies that provide the modern context for, nursing practice. We need to understand the reasons why nurses are being asked to work in particular ways. It is not an exploration of nursing theories or philosophies that have guided nursing from *within* the profession. It is rather a discussion of the *external* policy decisions that are affecting the profession now.

These external policy decisions now include further emphasis on 'patient and public engagement' (PPE) and the links between sustainability, climate change and health.

In Chapter 3, 'The elements of working together: structure, process and culture', we will discuss those things that have to be in place if successful working together is to be achieved. These are what we may call the three elements of structure, process and culture. There will be an emphasis on culture particularly because it is this element that might be more under the influence of individuals and groups of nurses to change.

Chapter 4, 'Interprofessional working: the doctor–nurse relationship and collaborative practice', will explore the nature of the working relationship of arguably the two dominant professions in the health service as an example of the sorts of issues that help or hinder collaborative working. Many of the examples are necessarily drawn from acute hospital care simply because this is where the research has been. However, there are lessons that can be applied to other care settings.

In Chapter 5, 'Teamwork', we will explore the nature of teamworking. Much of the literature is drawn from the world of business, leadership and management but applies equally to healthcare. This will examine what the difference is between a team and a group, what an effective team may look like and the roles that individuals may bring to a successful team.

Chapter 6, 'Understanding people, understanding yourself', takes a more individual, psychological perspective to explore how to go about understanding others, how we gain impressions and interact with others, and the identification of some current ideas such as emotional intelligence (introduced in earlier chapters) in an attempt to guide personal reflection and development.

Chapter 7, 'Interprofessional education for collaborative practice', will discuss interprofessional education, as this is seen as a way of enhancing practice as well as the educational experience of professionals.

Learning features

Learning from reading text is not easy. For some it does not constitute learning at all! Therefore, to provide variety and to assist with the development of reflective and critical thought, this book contains reflective tasks, case studies and further reading to enable you to participate in your own learning. There will be material in the book to reflect upon. Other tasks may direct you to the clinical environment, other people or your own knowledge and values. There is always the internet and online resources. You will need to develop your own study skills and 'learn how to learn' to get the best from the material. The book cannot provide all the answers – the subject is too big and developments are too fast-moving to be included. The book therefore provides a frame-work for your learning. You will have to fill in many of the inevitable gaps. Therefore, we encourage you to develop your learning skills, learn how to access and analyse material, and be literate with information technology.

Activities

Throughout the book you will find activities in the text that will help you to make sense of, and learn about, the material being presented by the authors.

Some activities ask you to reflect on aspects of practice, or your experience of it, or the people or situations you encounter. Reflection is an essential skill in nursing, and it helps you to understand the world around you and often to identify how things might be improved. Other activities will help you develop key skills, such as your ability to think critically about a topic in order to challenge received wisdom, or your ability to research a topic and find appropriate information and evidence, and to make decisions using that evidence in often difficult and time-pressured situations. Finally, communication and working as part of a team are core to all nursing practice. Some activities will ask you to carry out group activities or think about your communication skills to help develop these.

All the activities require you to take a break from reading the text, think through the issues presented and carry out some independent study, possibly using the internet. Where appropriate, there are sample answers presented at the end of each chapter, and these will help you to understand more fully your own reflections and independent study. Remember, academic study will always require independent work: attending lectures will never be enough to be successful on your programme, and these activities will help to deepen your knowledge and understanding of the issues under scrutiny and give you practice at working on your own.

You might want to think about completing these activities as part of your personal development plan (PDP) or portfolio. After completing the activity, write it up in your PDP or portfolio in a section devoted to that particular skill. Then look back over time to see how far you are developing. You can also spend more time on the activities for a key skill that you have identified a weakness in, which will help build your skill and confidence in this area.

Chapter 1

Working with other people

Draft NMC Standards for Pre-registration Nursing Education

This chapter will address the following draft competencies:

Domain: Professional values

1. All nurses must practise confidently according to *The Code: Standards of conduct, performance and ethics for nurses and midwives* (NMC, 2008), and other ethical and legal codes, recognising and responding appropriately to situations in day-to-day practice.
4. All nurses must work with patients, carers, groups, communities and other organisations, taking account of their strengths and needs. They must aim to empower people to make choices and decisions to promote self-care and safety while managing risk and promoting health and wellbeing.

Domain: Leadership, management and team working

1. All nurses must demonstrate leadership skills and support and improve the wellbeing and healthcare experience of people, communities and populations through quality improvement and strategic development.

Draft Essential Skills Clusters

This chapter will address the following draft ESCs:

Cluster: Care, compassion and communication

1. As partners in the care process, people can trust a newly registered graduate nurse to provide collaborative care based on the highest standards, knowledge and competence.

By first progression point:

ii. Works within limitations of the role and recognises own level of competence.
iv. Shows respect for others.
v. Is able to engage with people and build caring professional relationships.

Draft Essential Skills Clusters continued

Cluster: Organisational aspects of care

11. People can trust the newly registered graduate nurse to safeguard children and adults from vulnerable situations and support and protect them from harm.

By first progression point:

ii. Shares information with colleagues and seeks advice from appropriate sources where there is a concern or uncertainty.

By entry to the register:

vi. Shares information safely with colleagues and across agency boundaries for the protection of individuals/the public.
viii. Works collaboratively with other agencies to develop, implement and monitor strategies to safeguard and protect individuals and groups who are in vulnerable situations.

Chapter aims

After reading this chapter you will be able to:

- work towards defining what 'working with other people' may mean;
- list and define the terms used, such as interprofessional, interdisciplinary, multiprofessional, multidisciplinary and collaborative practice;
- identify the key stakeholders involved in 'working with other people';
- begin to think critically about communication in healthcare.

Introduction

The title of this book outlines two important ideas. The first is the need for nurses to work with other professionals and the second is to work with 'people'. It is the case that, depending on the work setting (a hospital ward, someone's home), these people get labelled as 'patients' and 'clients'. This book will refer to 'people' and where the context demands it, *client* and *patient* may be used. However, the important point here is that nursing work is *'working with other people'*, be they professionals, non-professionals, patients, clients, families or children.

Therefore, before we begin to understand the issues that arise from 'working with other people', we need to think first about what we mean by that phrase. In all likelihood, you will already have experience of working with others either at school, college or in the workplace. You may therefore already have some understanding from experience of what this means. However, as Chapter 2 on policy and context outlines, 'working with other people' in the National Health Service (NHS) is something quite complex. Therefore we will need to understand who these people are, their roles and the degree of their involvement. Some people are consulted (or told) only on the odd occasion about care decisions, while others are involved directly in such things as assessment of care needs and implementing care on a daily basis. Some are professionals but many are not. This chapter will identify the key 'stakeholders' (i.e. the people who have an interest in health services), outlining their involvement, and will also introduce the concepts of interprofessional working and collaborative practice. We will also discuss other terminology in common use.

We will also need to understand factors that help, and factors that hinder, working together. There are *processes* (the many ways we work together, including our professional codes of conduct that we use to define our practice, our use of language and the knowledge base from which we draw) and *structures* (which includes physical space, equipment and skills mix – e.g. the ratio of registered nurses to care assistants) that define how we work.

Alongside structure and process is culture. Chapter 3 will address this in more detail.

Before we explore in any detail who are the people in the term 'people', we need to be clear about the settings and terms used. Many nurses work in a public sector organisation, the NHS, but not exclusively so. You need to realise that the setting in which healthcare is delivered may have implications for how that care is accessed by people and delivered by professionals, and you need to know the key terms used by many professionals, theorists and commentators that refer to these settings.

Public, private and third sector

Much of what applies in an NHS setting (the *public* sector) also applies in an independent setting (or the *private* sector). The general public seeks healthcare from a wide variety of sources and providers, and it may be the case that registered nurses in the future will work in many more contexts and with a variety of employers. This may affect the way we work in quite dramatic ways. There is also the *informal care* sector, which may be overlooked but which provides the bulk of caring services. This includes family – usually women, and less often friends or neighbours.

A new and emerging term could also be included – the *third sector*, which relates to independent organisations that deliver care (sometimes on behalf of the NHS). Some of these organisations are charities and voluntary bodies that are increasingly involved in health and social care delivery.

Activity 1.1 *Evidence-based practice and research*

The terms 'public sector' and 'private sector' are often used when discussing healthcare (as well as education and social care). You may already be familiar with what these terms mean from reading newspapers, listening to the radio or watching television.

Check your understanding by:

*   defining what they mean;
*   thinking how this might affect the way you could be asked to work in each sector.

(Hint: How are staff educated and trained? How is success measured?)

A brief outline answer is given at the end of the chapter.

In this activity, you may have come across the following definitions:

* **Public sector**
  government and its activities: the portion of a nation's affairs, especially economic affairs, that is controlled by government agencies.
  (http://encarta.msn.com)

The public sector is that part of economic and administrative life that deals with the delivery of goods and services by and for the government, whether national, regional or local/municipal.

(http://en.wikipedia.org/wiki/Public_sector)

- **Private sector**

privately owned part of economy: the part of a free market economy that is made up of companies and organizations that are not owned or controlled by the government.

(http://encarta.msn.com)

That portion of the economy composed of businesses and households, and excluding government.

(http://en.wikipedia.org/wiki/Private_sector)

- **Third sector**

The UK government sees the 'third sector' as those organisations that are neither private or public. The government defines the third sector as *non-governmental organisations which are value-driven and which principally reinvest their surpluses to further social, environmental or cultural objectives. It includes voluntary and community organisations, charities, social enterprises, cooperatives and mutuals.* It remains to be seen how this sector will impact in the delivery of healthcare. An example that may increasingly be relevant to health is that of 'social enterprises', which *are businesses with primarily social objectives whose surpluses are principally reinvested for that purpose in the business or in the community, rather than being driven by the need to maximise profit for shareholders and owners* (www.cabinetoffice.gov.uk/third_sector/about_us/index.asp).

Working with other people

'Working with other people' means working with service *providers* (who are often, but not exclusively, professionals) and service *users*, in a collaborative way. It may mean the different professional groups working together (interprofessional), sharing expertise and information. It may also mean blurring roles and educational practices.

At first, it seems obvious to understand what collaborative, interprofessional practice may mean, but as is often the case, first appearances may be deceptive. Therefore, there is a need to define what we mean, and a good start may be to identify who the 'people' are. The 'working with' could be taken to mean *collaboration*, but as we will discuss, this may not always be the case.

Scenario 1.1

You arrive at work at the beginning of a morning shift on a busy surgical ward. You hang up your coat and walk towards the office. As you walk down the corridor you greet Maureen the housekeeper and nod to Dr McCormack (Joe) who is looking intently at an X-ray with a senior colleague, the imposing figure of Mr Downs, one of the surgical consultants. Joe is not long out of medical school and is still settling into his first clinical role. Mr Downs seems to be waiting for Joe's opinion on the X-ray he has in his hand. On entering the office you note that you are one of the first to arrive. Sandra, the care assistant, is sitting down and smiles warmly at you. In the ward there is a quiet hum of activity. David, the physiotherapist, pops his head around the door to see if the charge nurse, Bob, is in the office. Sandra mentions in passing that 'management' are keen to increase the returns on the patient

Scenario 1.1 continued

satisfaction survey and that staff are being 'encouraged to engage the patients in this process'. She smiles broadly as she quotes from the memo.

A cursory glance at the above indicates the scale of the issue. In one short walk down a corridor you have met:

- a housekeeper;
- a junior doctor;
- a consultant surgeon;
- a care assistant;
- a physiotherapist.

Also, in one short exchange with Sandra, two other groups of people have come into focus – 'management' and patients. You know that as the day progresses you will have to deal with many of these people in some shape or form.

You are a Community Psychiatric Nurse (CPN) visiting Mr and Mrs Jones in their own house. Following deterioration in his health Mr Jones has been anxious, losing weight and getting depressed. Mrs Jones had phoned her GP, Dr Singh, during the night following a panic attack. Dr Singh will be joining you to discuss the management of the immediate situation.

Scenario 1.2

Mr Jones has a long-standing chronic illness which, now he is in his eighties, has recently deteriorated. Mrs Jones, who is retired, is his only carer.

During the meeting you review case notes from Mr Jones's hospital consultant, and the assessment of the couple's social care needs. There is a need to ensure that a care package is in place to support the couple in their own home. Social services will need to be involved and you consider someone with talking therapy or counselling skills. During the discussion you ask about any other immediate family.

As in the previous scenario, you will see that there are five professionals (nurse, social worker, counsellor, therapists and doctor), at least two 'agencies' (social services, primary care) and a reference to another professional (hospital consultant). In addition, Mr and Mrs Jones will need support from any family and care support workers for social and personal care needs.

In both cases, you will note that working interprofessionally to provide a comprehensive care package for people is absolutely central. Reflect on the care needs: they will be personal, physical, social and psychological. Mrs Jones, as a carer, will have her own care needs in this situation. What would be the issues facing her?

A hospital, a general practice surgery, a primary care-based Community Mental Health Team (CMHT), or a supported living environment for people with learning disabilities, will all involve a large number of staff who keep the whole organisation functioning. Many will be, to borrow a term from the restaurant industry, 'front of house', i.e. visible. Others will be working behind the scenes. All, however, will contribute to the organisation's (hopefully) smooth running and the integration of care for patients and clients.

It is advisable that you know who these people are and how they work. Your future care role will involve the coordination of services and the planning of patient care. You cannot do this without knowing what other people do.

Therefore, the definition of working with other people used in this text means the broad spectrum of everyone involved in the process of healthcare receipt and delivery.

Interprofessional and collaborative practice

Many of those you will be in contact with are *professionals* working within *disciplines* and you will hear the terms 'interprofessional' and 'multiprofessional' and 'inter-disciplinary' and 'multidisciplinary'. These terms need clarification because they are used sometimes interchangeably in the literature. As a professional, it is important that your use of language is as precise as it can be to convey what we are trying to say or describe. Having said that, professionals and academics are often not the best at being clear! Leathard (1994, p5) hints at this lack of clarity by referring to a 'terminological quagmire'.

One way to think about this is to look at the prefixes 'inter' and 'multi'. 'Inter' is used to form an adjective meaning 'between (or among) people, things or places'. 'Multi' simply means 'many'. Therefore, multiprofessional working is not the same as interprofessional working, although the terms are often used as if they are. 'Interprofessional' indicates some level of *collaboration* or working together, whereas 'multiprofessional' should mean that there are two or more professions involved, but not necessarily in a *collaborative* manner.

Similarly, 'profession' and 'discipline' may not be the same.

There is a great deal of literature on what constitutes a profession, including debates on whether nursing can call itself a profession or should be classified by others as a profession. While this debate is interesting in its own right, for the purposes of understanding the nature of interprofessional working, the literature published by the Department of Health (and many other organisations such as the Cochrane Collaboration, who use the term 'professions allied to medicine') seems to accept that this means a *specialist occupational work group*. There is often tacit acceptance of traditional views that understand medicine, law, nursing, midwifery, social work, teaching, physiotherapy, etc. to be regarded as professions.

Discipline

The word 'discipline' comes from the Latin *disciplina* – 'instruction given to a learner' (http://encarta.msn.com/):

- **training to ensure proper behaviour**: the practice or methods of teaching and enforcing acceptable patterns of behaviour;
- **order and control**: a controlled orderly state, especially in a class of school children;
- **calm, controlled behaviour**: the ability to behave in a controlled and calm way even in a difficult or stressful situation;
- **conscious control over lifestyle**: mental self-control used in directing or changing behaviour, learning something, or training for something;
- education **activity** or **subject**: a subject or field of activity, e.g. an academic subject.

It is usually the first point and the fifth point above that we mean when we talk about a discipline.

'To discipline' (as a verb) may refer to the way we train ourselves and others to produce a set of character traits or behaviours in a specified group of people. The last point suggests that 'a discipline' (as a noun) is an educational/academic subject or an activity.

Disciplines can be seen to operate *within* professions, i.e. within the profession of medicine it is arguable that there are the separate disciplines of surgery, psychiatry, anaesthetics and others. In nursing, the separate disciplines are identified as 'branches' – adult, mental health, child and learning disabilities. These will become 'fields of practice' from September 2011. We may also think of disciplines such as critical care, community psychiatric nursing and school nursing.

We need to note that there is argument over these classifications. So, for example, whether school nurses or health visitors see themselves as a 'discipline' or a separate 'profession' is an argument that has been debated for many years. Currently, health visiting and school nursing are very much part of nursing, but at a specialist level. Both groups have to be on the first part of the register (as 'ordinary' registered nurses) before undertaking further study to be registered as health visitors and school nurses as specialists. There are those who argue (Houston and Cowley, 2002) that health visiting, with its roots in public health (Craig and Smith, 1998), is a separate discipline from nursing and is underpinned by a social model of health as opposed to a medical model of nursing. This suggests that these groups have a separate *role identity* and may define their work very differently. Some health visitors and school nurses have suggested that the nursing title should be abandoned, but others see themselves very much as nurses. Discussions continue on this topic.

This debate illustrates that the use of words to describe an occupational group or activity is not just an academic exercise. Staff groups take very seriously the titles and words used to describe what they do.

You may come across the term 'multidisciplinary team' in healthcare. Often this means the same as several professions working together, each providing their own insights and knowledge, but coming together in case conferences to share knowledge in the review of a patient's progress.

The differing professions may work in the same clinical setting, but they may still keep within their own clearly defined role boundaries. For example, think about a patient's medications management. For simplicity's sake, the doctor prescribes, the pharmacist dispenses and the nurse administers. This is a huge generalisation and oversimplification, but the point is that each profession has its own specific area of expertise when dealing with the same patient's drugs. In reality, there has always been a blurring of these roles and, with the advent of experienced professionals who take the title and role of 'non-medical prescribers', the blurring of role boundaries has become official. However, this simple description of medicines management is not 'multidisciplinary'.

Professionals working in a shared way, however, has not been seen as a natural state of affairs.

Stephen Ladyman MP, Parliamentary Under Secretary of State for Community, argued:

> The(re) are . . . *reasons why we must raise our standards of care and create a fully professional and respected (social workers) workforce. And why we must ensure that we break down barriers to good care provision and get rid of professional silos and negative attitudes that stop care professionals working together for common goals.*
>
> (25 March 2004)

The image of a 'silo' suggests that professionals may work separately whether they are in multidisciplinary teams or not. This may result in poor communication and breakdowns in care provision. The debates raised by school nurses and health visitors mentioned above illustrate how differing groups of workers see their values as being possibly quite different from those of a similar group of health workers.

Thus, the discussions about whether nursing is a 'discipline' or a 'profession' may be interesting in learned journals, but we only raise it here as you will come across many terms that are used to describe how the occupational groups work together. The real point is not what they call themselves but the level of collaboration and integration. Therefore, it may seem somewhat academic in healthcare practice whether one refers to professions and/or disciplines. Language use is dynamic and terms vary in meaning depending on who is using them and when they are being used. Pietroni (1992) identifies that there are at least 11 differing subsets of language used by the professions to describe themselves. This means that there is a good chance that we will not agree or understand each other when we come together to collaborate.

In universities the academic disciplines may be referred to as *subjects*, e.g. Physics, Geography, Engineering, Law and Nursing, hence confusing the picture even more.

Concept summary

Interprofessional/interdisciplinary

One definition of 'interprofessional working' is that of professionals *collaborating* to work together more effectively to improve the quality of patient care.

Multiprofessional/multidisciplinary

People from different professions are involved but this does not imply collaboration.

Thinking about the patient's perspective, what do you think their priorities are? Is the label really important? It may be that if I have an appointment to see a doctor, I have certain expectations about what the doctor can do. Am I concerned there is a debate about whether he or she is a discipline or a profession? Two reports (see the following boxes, 'Patients love our nurse-run surgery' and 'Patients prefer nurses') suggest that patients are not hide-bound to tradition or overly concerned about professional titles. Going to see a GP or a nurse practitioner may be equally acceptable to patients.

CASE STUDY: 'PATIENTS LOVE OUR NURSE-RUN SURGERY'

Doctors' leaders say that a nurse may be the first point of contact for many patients visiting surgeries – but how does this work in practice?

The Meadowfields Practice is probably the only one of its type in the country. Most surgeries have 'GP principals' – family doctors who run the show, and pay the salaries of other professionals, such as practice nurses, receptionists and managers. However, at Meadowfields, there is a 'Nurse principal' – Catherine Baraniak.

According to the British Medical Association (BMA), her practice may become a model for the surgery of the future. A shortage of doctors means that they have to work smarter, not just harder, and that patients with conditions that could be helped by the nurse should not necessarily take up their time.

Catherine Baraniak opened the surgery in August 1998. It offers its 3,000 patients a choice of seeing either a nurse or a GP. Most choose the nurse. She can order routine tests, give health advice, carry out some treatments, and even refer the patient on to a consultant if test results suggest that should be the case. At that point, the BMA had a slightly different view of what nurses should be allowed to do.

CASE STUDY continued

She told BBC News Online: 'They sent out a guidance note to hospital consultants saying that they should not accept patient referrals from nurses.' However, over the past few years, she has gradually won hospital specialists over to the once-heretical notion that a nurse could do all these things. And in a survey of southern Derbyshire practices, in terms of patient satisfaction, Meadowfields tops the lot.

Unlike many surgeries, you do not have to phone for an appointment here – just turn up. Ms Baraniak said: 'We feel it's the right thing to do, to offer a choice between seeing a nurse and the GP.

'Of the 35% who choose the GP, we would say that about half of them make the right choice. Many of them think that nurses can't do things like write sicknotes – when in fact we can, we just have to give them to the GP to sign.'

Source: http://news.bbc.co.uk, Thursday, 28 February 2002.

CASE STUDY: PATIENTS PREFER NURSES

Patients are often more satisfied when they see a nurse than a GP during a consultation at a doctor's surgery. Nurses have also been shown to save the NHS money when they take on tasks traditionally carried out by GPs.

A study, published in the British Medical Journal (Chau Shum et al., 2000), focused on approximately 1,800 patients with minor illnesses who attended one of five GP surgeries in South East London and Kent. Patients who saw a nurse gave them a 78.6% satisfaction rating, compared with doctors who were given a 76.4% score.

One of the key reasons why nurse consultations were more popular was the fact that they were able to spend more time with patients – an average of two minutes longer than GPs. The researchers said their findings indicated that nurses were able 'to offer a clinically effective service'. However, they warned that nurses might struggle to cope with rarer conditions.

The findings were echoed by a separate study (Kinnersley et al., 2000), which compared consultations given by GPs and nurse practitioners in 10 general practices in South Wales and South West England. It found that patients consulting nurse practitioners were generally more satisfied with their care, having been given longer consultations and more information about their illnesses.

Source: http://news.bbc.co.uk, Thursday, 13 April 2000.

Agency

The term 'agency' is also used frequently. You will have seen 'recruitment agency', 'environment agency' or reference made to social service or healthcare 'agencies'. For example, *Every Child Matters* is a UK government initiative run by the Department for Children, Schools and Families (DCSF). It attempts to provide children's services and aims to work with a wide range of partners, including government departments, non-departmental public bodies and other agencies:

> Children's social services seek to promote the well-being of children in need and looked-after children. They work in partnership with key agencies, service users and the community, to pursue continuous improvements in quality, efficiency and cost through best value.

> (www.everychildmatters.gov.uk)

Therefore, an 'agency' can be understood as a term with broad meaning. It may or may not be government run and funded; it is an organisation to provide a service employing a range of professional and non-professional staff. Social services, for example, may have 'adoption agencies' and this term will be used explicitly in the title of that department, but other 'agencies' consulted in the care of children may be a GP practice. As with other terms already discussed, the meaning is often known to those using it at the time but is not always clear to those new to understanding how organisations work together.

Collaboration

We have noted above that, in discussions of what interprofessional working may mean, the word 'collaboration' is often used. *Collaboration*, as Hornby and Atkins (2000) state, may be:

> A relationship between two or more people, groups or organisations, working together to define and achieve a common purpose. At delivery level, collaboration takes place between the people who need some kind of help and the people who provide it, and between the providers.

> (p7)

Biggs (1997) states that collaboration involves working together to achieve something that neither agency (or profession) could achieve alone. This definition highlights the importance of working together, suggesting that certain patient outcomes could not be achieved if people did not come together.

Collaborative practice, as proposed by Barrett et al. (2005), is about:

> [a] common purpose of developing mutually negotiated goals achieved through agreed plans and monitored and evaluated according to agreed procedures. This requires pooling of knowledge and expertise to facilitate joint decision making based upon shared professional viewpoints.

> (p18)

It needs to be emphasised that Hornby and Atkins use the word 'people' and write 'that need help.' The Barrett statement does not explicitly mention the people who need help as being part of the process, but this could be read implicitly into the definition. Terminology is important here as this brings to our attention that this is not just about how paid professionals or disciplines or occupational groups work together. This is also about how the people (users and carers) are brought into the process rather then being seen as passive recipients of services.

Barrett et al. (2005) go on to state that *interprofessional working* means the same thing as collaborative practice, which is:

the process whereby members of different professions and/or agencies work together to provide integrated health and/or social care for the benefit of service users.

(p10)

Again, note that the 'service user' in this latter definition is not explicitly engaged in the decision-making process. Hence, the definition may be inadequate in the context of the current NHS, where the aim from the Department of Health is that the public are central to decision making. Patients therefore need to be considered as partners in decision making and care delivery rather than just being recipients of it.

Also, this does not say *how* (or *what*) this process is. We need to think about how groups actually work together, whether and how they share roles, knowledge, information, education and training. It does not explicitly discuss hierarchy or teamworking. The process therefore could be quite varied.

For a discussion on and definitions of the various terms, see Day (2006) who uses Rawson's (1994) 'categorisations'. The suggestion here is that you can combine the terms in Table 1.1 to explore any aspect of working with other people. This also illustrates the complex nature of the concepts we are discussing. So, when analysing and describing a working situation, pick out a word from each category that most accurately describes what is going on. Thus, is a clinical work group inter/professional/work, or are we talking about multi/occupational/teamwork? We will return to the notion of 'teamworking' in Chapter 5.

Does any of this matter? Possibly it does not for those delivering the actual care to patients. However, as we will see in the next chapter, those who are directing and designing health services are concerned about what we call work groups and the analysis of how they work together. Therefore, the use of terms to describe what they are talking about is important. In your work you will hear these terms and you need to be able to unpick what people actually mean when they use them.

Table 1.1: 'Categorisations' to describe working with other people.

Category	Terms
Category 1: 'Problematic' associations	• Inter (between, among) • Multi (many) • Trans (across)
Category 2: Grouping	• Professional • Occupational • Disciplinary • Sectoral (see public/private/third sectors) • Agency (an organisation providing a service)
Category 3: Focus of operation	• Work • Teamwork • Collaboration • Cooperation • Integration

Interprofessional

A common term used is *interprofessional*. Day (2006, p9) clarifies the definition of 'interprofessional' by stating:

> *Persons belonging to a profession, relating between and among each other, for the mutual benefit of those involved.*

We should note that, when discussing 'interprofessional working', we must not overlook the fact that the user of the service could be involved in the process. The above definition does not explicitly state this to be the case as it addresses inter*professional* working. One definition may lead to another. What does 'relate' mean?! Again, this may seem pedantic as we are picking over the meaning of words, but there is a reason for this. In *Alice in Wonderland*, Lewis Carroll has Humpty Dumpty asserting that *when I use a word, it means what I want it to mean.* This assertion, that words can mean anything that the user wishes them to mean, is a recipe for confusion. You *may* define a word as you want, but you can't *use* a word to mean whatever you want if you expect others to agree with you. Go to a restaurant and try to have water by asking the waiter for Coke. We need shared meanings and definitions if we are to agree that we are talking about the same thing. So, if we cannot define and agree on what 'interprofessional' working is, how will we know whether to promote it, develop it, measure it or evaluate its success?

Key stakeholders

Many people are not 'professionals' at all, but they perform roles that are vital – the cleaners, domestic and housekeeping workers and administrative staff, e.g. ward clerks. Much of the literature and policy documents covering this field mentions inter-professional collaboration, but it is important that we include other groups who are directly or indirectly involved in the care of people, not the least of whom are patients, clients, users and carers. Their needs and interests are imperative and the Department of Health (DH 1994, 1998b, 2000a – *The NHS Plan*, plus the more recent *Patient and Public Involvement in Health* (DH, 2007)) has recognised their role in healthcare delivery.

Concept summary: Stakeholders

A stakeholder can be defined as **Somebody or something with direct interest:** *a person or group with a direct interest, involvement, or investment in some-thing, e.g. the employees, shareholders, and customers of a business concern* (http://uk.encarta.msn.com/dictionary). 'Stakeholder' has many definitions in law and management but is also used in health and social care. It can be used as a general term to denote a large group of people 'who are (or might be) affected by any action taken by an organisation or group'. Examples are parents, children, customers, owners, employees, associates, partners, contractors, suppliers, and people who are related or located nearby.

In a healthcare organisation this means the staff who organise and deliver care as well as the user of the service. These people have a 'stake' in the outcome of any service delivery. They are affected by how the organisation works. They also affect the process due to their inputs into the service or the way they are consulted in service delivery. Their inputs may be the physical work they do, the education they provide, the management of the finances or the way they organise delivery.

- You may begin to think that some stakeholders are 'more equal than others'. Consider whose voice gets heard when care delivery is decided.

Stakeholders are those with an interest in the performance of the organisation. They affect, and are affected by, the decisions made. We will list who these stakeholders are, but in no order of importance:

- physiotherapists;
- occupational therapists;
- social workers;
- dieticians;
- speech therapists;
- podiatrists;
- chiropodists;
- pharmacists;
- doctors – consultants, registrars, senior and house officers, GPs;
- radiographers;
- audiologists;
- nurses (mental health, adult, child and learning disabilities), consultant nurses, specialist nurses;
- nurse practitioners in emergency care;
- cognitive behavioural therapists;
- psychologists;
- counsellors;
- health visitors;
- midwives;
- dentists;
- dental nurses;
- paramedics;
- emergency care practitioners;
- management – all levels;
- education and training staff.

Other staff who support in providing care include:

- ambulance technicians;
- care assistants or associate practitioners;
- auxiliaries;
- ward clerks;
- receptionists;
- cleaners;
- housekeepers;
- administrators;
- porters;
- IT and technical support;
- voluntary and independent agency staff.

This is not an exhaustive list. In the future, in your role as a registered practitioner, you will need to understand what many of these people do, what their skills are and how they interact with nursing staff (see Scenario 1.3). You will already have an idea of the role of some of these occupational groups but check your understanding. For example, what is the difference between a counsellor and a psychologist? What is a cognitive behavioural (CB) therapist? How does an ambulance technician differ from a paramedic and how does a paramedic differ from an emergency care practitioner – what can you expect from each of them? How are they educated, what client groups do they work with, what expertise do they bring, when are you likely to come across them in practice?

And, last but not least, patients may be seen as the most important stakeholders of all!

Scenario 1.3

Sammy Lee is ten years old and has Down's syndrome. He also has a congenital heart condition that now requires hospitalisation for assessment, investigations and treatment. Sammy lives with his parents and has been exhibiting challenging behaviour. The nurse who will admit Sammy will have to collaborate with a range of professionals: the cardiac consultant and his or her medical team, the learning disabilities services, radiographers, children's nurses, pharmacists, anaesthetists and operating department staff.

Therefore, this nurse will need to draw upon knowledge of children, learning disabilities and cardiac surgery in addition to working interprofessionally with a wide range of staff.

Healthcare professionals are often educated to degree level, i.e. as graduates, to gain entry onto a professional register. Of the list above, can you identify a missing healthcare group and can you identify which group is not educated to graduate level? What advantages (if any) does a graduate level of education bring to a professional group?

One delineation between the health professional groups is that of:

- medicine
- professions 'allied to medicine' (PAMs).

Activity 1.2   *Critical thinking*

The Cochrane Collaboration explicitly uses the term *'professionals allied to medicine'* (www.cochrane.org).

The Cochrane Collaboration is an international not-for-profit and independent organisation, dedicated to making up-to-date, accurate information about the effects of healthcare readily available worldwide. It produces and disseminates systematic reviews of healthcare interventions and promotes the search for evidence in the form of clinical trials and other studies of interventions.

This organisation issued guidelines that suggested: Professions allied to medicine, such as nurses, midwives and dieticians, can effectively incorporate clinical guidelines to improve patient care.

*The issuing of clinical guidelines to nurses, midwives, dieticians and other health-care professionals allied to medicine may reduce variations in practice and improve patient care. This review found that, despite limited research, there is some evidence that guidelines can improve care and that professional roles can be substituted effectively, **for instance a nurse can perform the function of a physician in certain circumstances**. Such interventions offer the possibility of reduced costs but further research is needed in all areas of this topic.*

(www.cochrane.org/reviews/en/ab000349.html, accessed 27 March 2007)

Users

Hornby and Atkins (2000) define two terms that may prove useful when considering who we are talking about: *user* and *faceworker*. They point out that those receiving care services are often known by a variety of words – patient, client, user, carer, resident. They argue that the terms are limiting in the context of the collaboration between professional groups (and care agencies) that is needed. By this they may mean that a 'patient' for a doctor is not the same as a 'client' for a social worker even when the 'patient' is the same person as the 'client' (see Scenario 1.4).

Scenario 1.4

Dr McCormack wishes to discharge his 'patient' from hospital and is involved in discussions to do this. The clinical environment is under pressure to admit more patients to meet targets, although in his heart Dr McCormack knows this is not why he wishes to discharge this patient. His patient has undergone medical and surgical intervention and has now recovered sufficiently to consider the next stage on the patient pathway. The patient is primarily seen and understood by the medical team as a 'case'. By recovery, Dr Jones is interested in such things as wound healing, and physiological parameters such as electrolyte balances, and the efficacy of a new drug prescription or the stability of the patient's vital signs of blood pressure, temperature and heart rate. As a holistically minded doctor, he also understands the psychological and social conditions of his patients. This means that he understands that his patient may be anxious about progress and depressed about complications that could well feature in prolonged hospitalisation.

Ms Goodyear is the social worker involved with the 'client' who needs discharging from hospital. Her client has certain social and welfare needs, and as an elderly pensioner is more than the sum of physiological processes. To Ms Goodyear, her work with social work clients involves 'making decisions to intervene, to protect vulnerable adults' (Barrett et al., 2005) and hence has a focus to ensure that before discharge her client has the care they require.

Are they discussing the same person? Is there a tension between the need to discharge a patient and meeting a client's social care needs? What do you think defines a person either as a patient or a client? (There are not necessarily right or wrong answers to these questions.)

Hornby and Atkins (2000) describe the term 'user' as:

the individual, couple, family or other group which uses help . . . emphasis(ing) an important underlying value; those that use help are defined on their own terms not in terms of the profession or agency providing help.

(p8)

In this manner we have turned the focus around, away from the professional or agency which defines people in particular ways and towards how users themselves may interpret their own situation and needs. This highlights a dynamic tension in understanding working with other people, i.e. how we define people may lead us to think in a way that the user themselves would not recognise or value. This also applies to the way we understand and define our co-workers.

Think of the difference between seeing someone as a 'patient', 'user' or even 'customer'. Why do you think travel companies now refer to passengers as 'customers'? What would be the implications of universities seeing students as customers as well as learners? What rights and privileges are associated with 'customer', 'user' or 'patient'?

Faceworkers

The distinction here is between those who work at 'ground' level rather than as support or managerial levels. From the users' standpoint, these are people they see 'face to face' when they need help. The 'faceworker' could, of course, be family, friends or the local community, or people who work in voluntary agencies. It is necessary to remind ourselves that this 'informal' sector provides a great deal (if not most) of the care needed. From a faceworker's perspective, they will find themselves within a matrix of agencies, professionals and non-professionals.

This terminology may assist with clarifying who the staff groups are, but for the purposes of this text the term 'nurse' will apply as the main 'faceworker' of focus. This is because you will not hear the term 'faceworker' in a clinical setting. You are studying to be a nurse and not a faceworker, although, of course, that is the role you will be undertaking.

Activity 1.3   *Critical thinking*

Adult branch nurses deal with *patients* in hospital. Mental health nurses have *clients*, as do learning disabilities nurses (who also have *residents*). Children's nurses deal with *families* and *children*.

- Does the use of these terms tell us something about the way we define people in our care? What is the difference between being a patient, client, resident, or child?

(Hint: Is this something to do with having certain 'rights'?)

An outline answer is given at the end of the chapter.

The 'user'

We have put users first to reflect the importance of this in the whole process. Your day-to-day experience may be talking with other professionals. Indeed, it is easy to miss the importance of communicating with users as much of your practice may involve large amounts of time in face-to-face contact with other faceworkers.

'Working with . . .' thus may mean interacting on a regular (usually, but not exclusively) face-to-face basis with others (users and faceworkers) to assess, plan, implement and evaluate care. This involves listening, discussing, valuing, participating, negotiating. Thus, this is not just about professionals working together or agencies working together. The exact nature of this will be explored in more detail later. However, it is worth looking at the user's experience in order to show how complex this may be and how nothing should be taken for granted. In Chapter 6 we will examine the ways we interact and form opinions of others and how this may shape who and what we believe people are.

CASE STUDY: COMMUNICATING WITH 'USERS'

A maternity department wanted to seek the views of their patients: the general questionnaire used by the Trust was of little help to them. They chose to use a method that had been used successfully by another hospital team on the Clinical Governance Development Programme. Patients are now given a (pre-paid) postcard when they are ready to leave hospital: it invites comments on the care they received. They are asked to return the card to a post-box on the ward – or send it back by Royal Mail. Community midwives remind patients to return them. Staff are pleased by patients' response to the cards. Positive comments have helped improve staff morale while criticisms are followed up promptly. Links between the hospital and the community have improved.

Lessons

- Don't 'reinvent the wheel' – adopt methods proven elsewhere.
- See what you can find out about techniques used by the others before you start to develop new ways of thinking.
- *Remember*, simple methods are often the best.

Source: www.cgsupport.nhs.uk.

This illustrates that the NHS is adopting many of the practices of the commercial and business world, i.e. patients may be seen to be customers from whom the service needs feedback to improve its service.

Research summary

Empirical studies into the nature of communication with users

The following is a small number of studies into nurse–patient interaction that describe the nature of this interaction in, not always, satisfactory ways. You need to understand that a small number of studies such as those that follow do not by themselves define the nature of nurse–patient interaction. This is a snapshot in a small number of selected clinical environments and therefore generalising to the wider population would be inappropriate. However, their inclusion here illustrates that assumptions need challenging about how a 'caring profession' interacts with patients.

McCann and McKenna (1993) examined the nature of nurse–patient touching in an elderly care setting in Northern Ireland. They suggested that most nurse–patient touch interactions were *instrumental* in nature. That is to say, patients were touched to perform a task, to get something done such as taking a blood pressure, almost as if the patients were seen as *objects*.

Kruijver et al. (2001) in a study of the nature of communication between nurses and simulated cancer patients conducted in Holland, suggested that over 60 per cent of nurses' talk was again *instrumental* in nature (means to an end, to get something done). *Affective* communication (i.e. that directed towards meeting emotional or 'feelings' needs) occurred, but did not get into actively discussing and exploring patients' feelings by *showing empathy, showing concern and optimism* (p722).

Wiman and Wikblad (2004) studied the encounters between nurses and trauma patients in an emergency department. The study was undertaken by observing ten nurses in a small number of care episodes. They argue that the nurses' verbal and non-verbal communication was poor, and that they adopted a wait-and-see policy. What they argue emerged from this was 'instrumental behaviour'.

> One of the caring aspects, [i.e.] being dedicated and having courage to be appropriately involved, could not be identified. Most encounters included several aspects of caring and uncaring, but the uncaring aspects predominated. The dominance of uncaring aspects indicates a lack of affective caring behaviour.
>
> (p422)

Kristiansen et al. (2005) report findings from a larger quantitative study (in Sweden) and they suggest that the feelings and attitudes that psychiatric nurses have towards their clients may reflect on the amount of time they spend with them. A key finding they report is that those who may be seen as the most vulnerable and dependent individuals received less staff attention and are the clients who spend the most time alone. They invoke the concept of *dehumanisation* to explain why certain clients receive less nursing attention.

Sorlie et al. (2006) argue (in a small-scale qualitative study, again in Sweden) that patients who reported satisfaction with care in an acute ward may still be vulnerable to compromises in care. They argue that healthcare staff should not be complacent upon receipt of patient satisfaction ratings.

Henderson et al. (2007) in Australia studied nurse–patient interactions and found that they were mostly friendly and informative. However, opportunities to develop closeness were limited. The major source of dissatisfaction was when patients perceived that nurses were not readily available to respond to specific requests. Patient satisfaction with the service is more likely to be improved if nurses can quickly adapt their work to accommodate patients' requests or, alternatively, communicate why these requests cannot be immediately addressed.

As stated above, great caution has to be exercised in transferring the results of the above studies to other settings or countries. However, the range of similarities directs us to critically examine the nature of our communication with users.

How nurses perceive other people (patients, professionals other nurses) will be explored later. As the above research suggests, it is important that we understand this process and that we analyse and are critical of how we interact with people.

Conclusion

The fact that there are many words to describe the nature of working relationships confuses the picture. Many policy makers and individuals use words in an *Alice in Wonderland* fashion, to mean whatever the individual wants them to mean. If you were to ask staff what 'interprofessional working' means, you will get a rich variety of answers. The use of the word 'client' as opposed to 'patient' has been a topic of debate because of the connotations associated with those words. Therefore, listen very carefully to the words being used, and ask yourself and others to clarify exactly what they mean when using the jargon. Part of your academic and professional development concerns your critical approach to the use of terminology.

CHAPTER SUMMARY

This chapter introduced the words and phrases commonly used by many people in discussions on 'working with others'. It is important to understand the wide range of words used and to grasp the fact that these words do not always mean the same thing. This can be very confusing, and not just to the novice! We began to look at what we mean by 'working with others' – to identify who these 'others' are. This may seem an obvious starting point, and it may also seem too obvious for discussion. Yet it may be an important step to recognise, and emphasise, that working with others means more than just developing collaboration with professional colleagues. It also means working 'with' patients and clients. This chapter also introduced the idea of 'collaboration'.

Activities: brief outline answers

Activity 1.1: Evidence-based practice and research (page 7)

- Simplistically, the public sector has a 'service to the public ethos' whereby providing that service takes precedence over commercial 'for profit' gain. Staff have traditionally traded relatively lower pay in return for job security and good pensions. The public to be served are viewed as patients and not customers. The sector itself paid for the education of staff. The government provided the funds for the service out of taxation. The private sector works in a competitive environment where the selling of the product for shareholder returns based on profits are paramount. Patients would be customers. Staff, beyond basic education, would be expected to fund their own development. If a service does not provide a profit or meet customer need, then it would not be provided. There is relatively little or no financial government support for activities.

This classic division, it is argued, is breaking down as private/public sector activities and philosophies get blurred.

Activity 1.2: Critical thinking (pages 18–19)

- In a Minor Injury unit a nurse may take a history of the patient's condition, conduct a clinical examination, order a clinical investigation (for example an X-ray), make a diagnosis, create a treatment plan, and in some cases prescribe medicines and discharge the patient, all without reference to a doctor. Implications may be that nurses will work towards being autonomous practitioners with greatly different educational needs, and that patients' expectations of what the NHS will provide will change.
- One explanation is based on the historical power of the medical profession to be the authoritative voice on all health matters and that this dominance is underpinned by the legal and professional framework that supports healthcare practice. See the General Medical Council's 'Good Medical Practice' (2006) www.gmc-uk.org/guidance/good_medical_practice/GMC_GMP.pdf

Activity 1.3: Critical thinking (page 20)

- Does the word 'patient' imply a traditional view of the doctor–patient relationship, one in which we defer to expertise and the direction of the professional? 'Client', on the other hand, is used in many other settings, often commercial 'for profit' settings, as well as social work and mental health. A client relationship implies more equality and one in which the client directs and collaborates with a professional to reach a mutually agreeable solution. 'Resident', of course, applies to hotels as well as care homes. Thus, the words used may be based on the assumed nature of the relationship between the people involved.

Knowledge review

Now that you've worked through the chapter, how would you rate your knowledge of the following topics?

	Good	Adequate	Poor
1. Public, private and third sectors.			
2. Interprofessional practice.			
3. Collaborative practice.			
4. Stakeholders.			

Where you are not confident in your knowledge of a topic, what will you do next?

Further reading

Barrett, G, Sellman, D and Thomas, J (2005) *Interprofessional Working in Health and Social Care*. Basingstoke: Palgrave Macmillan, especially Chapter 1.

Day, J (2006) *Interprofessional Working*. Cheltenham: Nelson Thornes, especially Chapter 2.

Hornby, S and Atkins, J (2000) *Collaborative Care: Interprofessional, interagency and interpersonal*, 2nd edition. Oxford: Blackwell Science.
This text discusses in detail the concept of collaborative care.

Williamson, G R, Jenkinson, T and Proctor-Childs, T (2010) *The Contexts of Contemporary Nursing*, 2nd edn. Exeter: Learning Matters.

Useful websites

www.dh.gov.uk This is one of the standard resources you should familiarise yourself with.

www.nice.org.uk Search for 'Patient and Public Involvement' programme.

The context: history and policy

Draft Essential Skills Clusters continued

By entry to the register:

vi. Provides safe and effective care in partnership with people and their carers within the context of people's ages, conditions and developmental stages.

Chapter aims

After reading this chapter you will be able to:

- understand the professional and the public policy context;
- have a view of the historical development of current policy;
- examine some of the factors that lead to the need to 'work together'.
- understand how contemporary policy focuses on collaborative working.

Introduction

The previous chapter introduced many terms that are used to describe working with other people. In order to be able to put it all in some historical context and to begin a critique of the direction in which this is going, we need to understand the 'drivers' of such initiatives. Several questions spring to mind:

- What are the policy statements that discuss the need to work more closely with others?
- What factors have led to the call for more interprofessional and collaborative working?
- What ideas do professionals have about the way they should work?
- In what ways are patients involved in this change?
- Who are the influential groups driving such policies?
- What has this meant for the way nurses now have to work?

You will need to ponder on these questions. Some answers are suggested below. However, you will possibly come up with your own ideas after reflecting on the various influences and actions you see in everyday clinical life.

After examining some government publications, we may begin to see that there is increasing pressure for professionals to work with a large number of stakeholder groups, to listen and respond to a variety of voices, and to act more like private-sector providers of services putting patients (as customers?) at the heart of professional practice, but not in a *paternalistic* (father/doctor/nurse knows best) kind of way.

What follows is an introduction to some of the main documents that have outlined the need for nurses to 'work with others'. It is not an exhaustive discussion. Public policy is a very complex subject, so an understanding of all the influences and theoretical perspectives would take several books in themselves. Therefore, the discussion here will introduce you to some of the ideas that support the policy towards interprofessional working or 'working with other people'.

A professional perspective

The Nursing and Midwifery Council (NMC), as the body responsible for public safety through the application of professional standards, has a view on how registered practitioners should conduct themselves. A good starting point to consider, therefore, is *The Code: Standards for conduct, performance and ethics* (NMC, 2008), which emphasises:

- care as the first concern, treating people as individuals, respecting their dignity;
- working with others to protect and promote the health and well-being of those in your care, their families, carers and the wider community;
- providing a high standard of practice and care at all times;
- being open and honest, and acting with integrity, upholding the reputation of the profession.

Activity 2.1   *Evidence-based practice and research*

- Look at the four points above and identify the key words.
- Give an example of 'maintaining dignity'.
- Explain what it means to 'act with integrity'.
- What is the reputation of the profession and how might that be brought into disrepute?

A brief outline answer is given at the end of the chapter.

From these four principles the NMC goes further, emphasising, for example:

- treating people as individuals, with dignity and kindness;
- respecting their confidentiality;
- collaborating with those in your care;
- gaining consent;
- maintaining professional boundaries;
- sharing information with colleagues;
- working effectively as a team;
- delegating effectively.

You will no doubt read *The Code* in detail during your course of study (**www.nmc-uk.org**). You will need to discuss each of the points above to interpret what they actually mean in practice. As a list they are 'hooray' words – meaning no one would disagree with them – but they may mean different things to different people. For example, how is dignity maintained for a Muslim wife? Are there cultural assumptions about what dignity means?

You may feel that some of these statements are self-evident – who would not approach someone with dignity and kindness? So, why has it been necessary to spell this out in detail? Have there been instances where lack of respect and dignity by nurses has come to the public's notice?

British society is in many areas multicultural, so patients will come from a wide variety of backgrounds. There will be differences of ethnicity, class, sexual orientation and, of course, gender. There will be differences in values, beliefs and attitudes. You will be exposed to people who you do not understand (and I do not mean simply their language) and with whom you have no 'connection'. They will not share your values or even want your care. Treating people with kindness, dignity and respect is easy when you like them as individuals, but you will, of course, be challenged by those who do not comply with your wishes or beliefs.

Working with others is as much about knowing yourself and your own values and issues, so as to cultivate awareness of your prejudices. If you think you do not have prejudices you may wish to reflect on your reasons for liking some people and not others.

The NMC also emphasises the team and collaborative nature of nursing, and thus recognises implicitly the NHS's concern with 'interprofessionalism'. This will be discussed later in this chapter.

Nursing care is delivered by a wide range of staff with different skills and abilities, and you will be asked to understand and work with this fact. Support workers will be working closely alongside registered nurses. In the future, assistant practitioners may become more numerous. You will need to understand the role and role boundaries very clearly. Read the case example for mental health support workers and think about how you would manage such developments to 'work effectively as a team'. What skills, knowledge and attitudes do you need to develop?

CASE STUDY: MENTAL HEALTH SUPPORT WORKERS

The following initiative is part of policy implementation. Mental health support workers are becoming more prevalent within community mental health teams and, until recently, they were Healthcare Assistants. However, there has been a development towards the STR (support, time and recovery) worker, which carries further responsibilities.

Community Psychiatric Nurses (CPNs) may work with STRs in a Community Mental Health Team (CMHT). Once the CPN has assessed a client's needs and written a clear care plan, community support workers (and STRs) will carry a small caseload and follow the interventions laid out in that care plan. These usually relate to social needs and include promoting recovery and social inclusion by way of helping with the general activities of daily living (taking people shopping, helping promote personal hygiene and getting people involved in therapeutic activities such as groups, etc.). There is also a role to play in monitoring mental health and reporting back any signs of relapse, all of which should be set out in the care plan.

The role of STR workers within the 'specialist' teams (Home Treatment, Assertive Outreach and Early Intervention) is similar, except that they 'team' nurse and do not carry an individual caseload. CPNs assess and work with people in crisis. When any significant risk has been seen to diminish, a CPN will then review the care plan and include interventions that STR workers can undertake. Such interventions are aimed squarely at recovery and relate to supporting individuals in whatever way possible to get better. Examples include getting people out of the home (to a café, group or to undertake other activities), promoting hygiene and social inclusion, helping with cooking and shopping, etc. In fact, the role is still developing and some of the work has been innovative and very creative. Exercise on prescription (offered by a growing number of GPs) has led to some STR workers working out in gyms with clients.

- In this case study you will need to understand the difference between *responsibility* and *accountability*. What are STRs responsible for? Who is accountable for their actions? Find out what these words mean.

The Royal College of Nursing (RCN) is a non-governmental body representing nurses' interests. The RCN (2006) states, as one of its principles of partnership in the document 'RCN principles: a framework for evaluating health and social care policy':

Collaborative decision making
Service providers and commissioners should demonstrate how they are actively and meaningfully engaging the public they serve and other stakeholders (such as staff and their representative bodies) in the design, delivery and evaluation of services regardless of the financial pressures.

(This is only one of eighteen elements in a framework of four main principles.)

Activity 2.2   *Critical thinking and group work*

Read the above RCN element, then think:

- Who are 'service providers'?
- Who are 'commissioners'?
- What is meant by design of services?
- Want is meant by delivery?
- What is meant by evaluation?

Discuss with others and then:

- identify how (if?) the public is engaged in design, delivery and evaluation of services;
- identify how staff are engaged in design, delivery and evaluation.

A brief outline answer is given at the end of the chapter.

Note that the RCN finds it necessary to state *regardless of the financial pressures.* We may reflect on such questions as: Why do you think they state this? How possible is it to act 'regardless of financial pressures'? Can you think of a situation in which you may have to take decisions about patient care with a view to the *cost* of that care?

Historical developments

Understanding how health and social care was organised in the early twentieth century is of interest for our discussion in comparing how far policy has changed and the impact that change has had on those who work for, and receive care from, a health service. It can be characterised as a shift away from fragmented, largely non-public sector provision where professional groups (and in health, especially medicine) delivered uncoordinated care across the country. So, for the pre-war period (before 1939) charities, civic bodies and independent professionals were charging for services without overarching national bodies and standards. The post-war changes meant an increasing role for the State (rather than professional groups) in the design, delivery and funding of health and social care.

The Beveridge Report (1942)

The 1942 report by William Beveridge set the foundation for the modern welfare state. After the Second World War (1939–45) the Labour government reforms (led by Prime Minister Clement Attlee) saw the introduction of the welfare state. Education reforms (especially the 1944 Education Act) and the establishment of the NHS in 1948 initiated a programme of public-sector State involvement in the health and well-being of UK citizens. This entailed the separation of health and social care (challenged by the Seebohm Report of 1968) with uniprofessional and local delivery of services. The professions (and semi-professions) had separate structures, education and practices. The 'post-war consensus' – a broad agreement between the Labour and Conservative governments (Elliot and Atkinson, 2007) – on public sector provision and the way it was delivered, remained until the end of the 1970s.

The 'post-war consensus' (the welfare state)

Sir William Beveridge's 1942 report, *Social Insurance and Allied Services* (not the most catchy title for what was a revolutionary report), laid the groundwork for the intervention of the state in the provision of education, employment and health in a way not experienced before. It was accepted by all political parties after the Second World War that the State had a legitimate role to play in key services to address poverty, poor education and ill health. The government was to fight Beveridge's five 'Giant Evils' of Want, Disease, Ignorance, Squalor and Idleness. This was not challenged until the 1970s, when Margaret Thatcher's Conservative government shifted public policy away from reliance on public sector provision and state intervention. It was thought that many of Britain's economic and social ills were based on too much interference from State bureaucracies. Elliot and Atkinson (2007) argue that Tony Blair adopted Thatcher's reforms and that for some policies took them further than the Conservative government would have.

1979–2007 government policy: the Thatcher–Blair consensus

Margaret Thatcher (the Conservative Prime Minister) was elected in 1979 and a key plank of her programme was the reform of public services. This was to place much greater emphasis on the concepts of public accountability, transparency of decision making and spending, *coherence between fragmented services* and the application of a *market consumerist philosophy*. There was to be more centralised control of public expenditure to achieve the goals of cost-effectiveness and promote patient and client choice. An internal market of purchasers and providers was created that shifted control from professionals to managers (Barrett et al., 2005). The Thatcher reforms also introduced the concept of *managerialism* – bringing private-sector practice into the public sector to tackle waste and inefficiency, giving power to managers to counteract trade unions and professionals, and to put the consumer at the centre of service provision.

Market consumerism: consumers or citizens?

A consumerist philosophy means that individuals place value on material possessions and consuming products (James, 2007). It is thought that this is the path to happiness and the good life. Market consumerism is a way of allocating resources according to people's willingness to pay for certain goods and services. It rests on the idea of the law of supply and demand – i.e. people will pay for a good up to the point where their ability to pay is matched to their desire to purchase. A supplier of the good will increase prices as long as they have consumers willing to pay. At the point where the price becomes too high for desire to have any effect, the consumer will not purchase and the supplier will not supply further.

This individual choice is collected into a market of others people's choices. The market then becomes the arbiter of supply and demand. It places consumer choice at the heart of production planning and delivery because it is accepted that the consumer knows best what is in their own interests.

Economically and politically it is a rebuttal of the idea that the State (social democratic, socialist or communist) is best placed to plan for the individual's needs. In health terms, this places the consumer at the heart of healthcare delivery planning. Patients in the post-war NHS did not have a choice of which hospital to attend when they were ill, and probably did not even think they could exercise a right of choice. Now, patients, in theory, are being offered choice about how, as well as where, they are to receive treatment. Thus, just as students are customers of education, so patients are customers of healthcare.

Taylor (2009) argued that too much emphasis has been placed on people being consumers rather than active citizens with responsibilities to society. Choice, thus, can be seen to be defined too narrowly, like the choice between two MP3 players. As active citizens, we would need to go beyond making mere choices to becoming active in our responsibilities to, for example, both our own health and the health care system.

The NHS was implicitly founded on the idea that the State (and the medical profession) knew best what health services are needed (*paternalism*). In a reaction to this, 'patient choice' can be seen as part of the wider cultural changes introduced by Margaret Thatcher's government's free-market consumerist philosophy. How far the 'customer is always right' mentality can actually be applied to health services is open to debate. The election of Tony Blair's government in 1997 did not radically alter this new (Thatcherist) view of public services. Indeed, public-sector reform, or '*modernisation*', was to gather pace. The range and number of legislative and policy initiatives has seen health and social care services restructured and reconfigured with increasing private sector involvement and ideas (e.g. Private Finance Initiative (PFI), Foundation Trust status). This has come to the point where the divide between public and private sector provision has become very blurred (Elliot and Atkinson, 2007).

Despite the changes to public sector provision started by Thatcher and continued by Blair and Brown, it could be argued that the State still has *the* key role. David Cameron's idea of the 'big society' further challenges the role of the state. The debate may be about what the mix of private sector, third sector and public sector involvement will look like, how government encourages the various agencies that provide services, and how it monitors the quality of provision and allocates funding. In addition to all of this is the question of the place of health and service professional groups' involvement in these changes.

The extent of government involvement can be illustrated by examining the budget. Figure 2.1 shows how much is being spent in one year on health-related issues.

The government thus plans to spend £119 billion on the health service, but if one takes a social model of health (i.e. one that accepts social determinants of health – employment, housing, etc.) then one has to add the £189 billion for social protection, £29 billion for housing and £31 billion for personal social services. Thus, out of a total of £671 billion, 'health' accounts for (119bn + 189bn + 29bn + 31bn) = £368 billion or 55 *per cent* of yearly expenditure!

The government increased spending on the NHS but in a context of a perception of structural difficulties in delivery. That is to say, despite changing the way the NHS works following huge inputs of money, many people wonder if patient care has actually improved (BBC, 2006a).

Reflect on stories in the national media concerning the NHS. Identify the main concerns that have been expressed.

As this is for your observation, there is no outline answer at the end of the chapter.

Figure 2.1: Government spending by function.

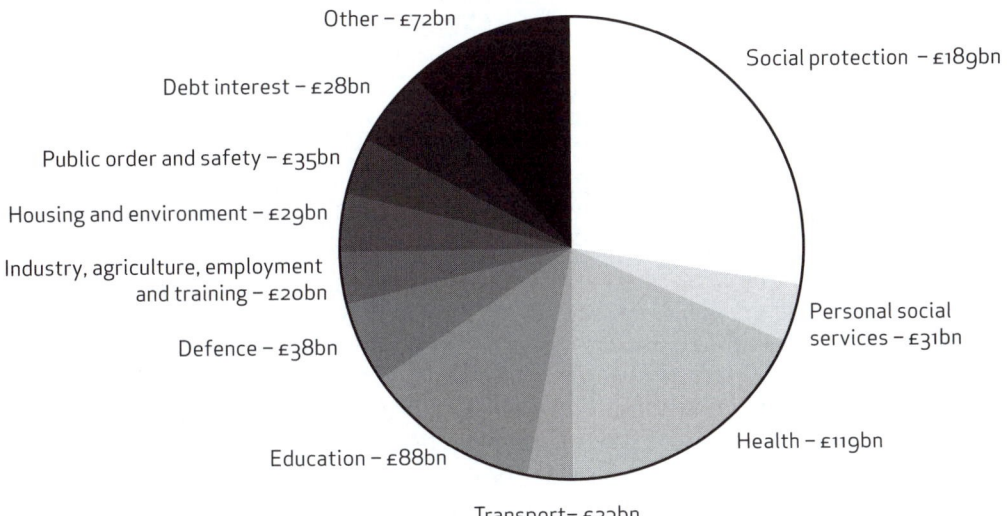

Other – £72bn
Social protection – £189bn
Debt interest – £28bn
Public order and safety – £35bn
Housing and environment – £29bn
Industry, agriculture, employment and training – £20bn
Defence – £38bn
Personal social services – £31bn
Education – £88bn
Health – £119bn
Transport– £23bn

Total managed expenditure – £671 billion.

Source: HM Treasury, 2009–10 near-cash projections.
Notes: Spending reclassified to functions compared to previous presentations and is now using methods specified in international standards. Other expenditure includes spending on general public services: recreation, culture, media and sport; international cooperation and development; public service pensions; plus spending yet to be allocated and some accounting adjustments. Social protection includes tax credit payments in excess of an individual's tax liability, which are now counted on AME, in line with OECD guidelines. Figures may not sum to total due to rounding.

The 'choice agenda'

Following on from the introduction of market-type reforms to public sector health services is the notion of giving back choice to people (who are now 'consumers of healthcare'), e.g. 'Choose and Book', where people are offered a choice of five independent, private or NHS hospitals in any area. In May 2007, *The Guardian* published a short series of commentaries from public policy commentators that are worth reflecting on. You may wish to think about what choice actually means, who has the ability to exercise choice and who is involved in providing choice options. Think particularly on Lord Patel's point about choice for ethnic minorities and the socially excluded. Is there also an issue about choice differences (access, availability, health priorities) between men and women?

Patrick Diamond (2007), a former special adviser in the Prime Minister's policy unit, has acknowledged that public service reform has not always been a success. He states that reform has come to mean a culture that focuses on targets, drawn up by centralised

CASE STUDY: THE GUARDIAN, MAY 2007: A MATTER OF CHOICE

Julian Le Grand, Professor of Social Policy, London School of Economics:

The choice agenda is not dead and nor should it be, because the whole purpose is to create incentives for improvement. Sometimes trusts do not put up information about the services they provide, so it's not there when doctors and patients search for it. Improving NHS information systems should sort this out. The Healthcare Commission survey that showed patients didn't regard choice as important was asking the wrong question. In effect, it said: 'Do you want a perfect TV or a choice of TVs?' People will always rank quality higher, but choice drives up quality and gives people what they want in the first place.

Ann Rossiter, Director, Social Market Foundation:

Choice, long the watchword for the reform of public services by New Labour, has fallen out of fashion. Gordon Brown does not seem particularly keen on the term, and his wariness is understandable. Choice was often presented, at least in the media, as a way of getting private-sector involvement in the public services, or alternatively, as reform for reform's sake. This was unfair. Choice is important because it offers the chance to empower service users – giving them control and, if it is used right, driving up standards. In these terms, choice has deep roots in progressive thinking. Nye Bevan, the creator of the NHS, argued that patients should be able to choose their GP. Choice is still important – but it must be choice in order to empower citizens in their relations with the public services.

Lord Kamlesh Patel, Head, Centre for Ethnicity and Health:

In a globalised consumer market, who can deny choice? But choice requires spare capacity, redundancy, higher costs. Nowhere is this more so than with healthcare. Research tells us patients don't want choice except when it isn't meaningful, when local services are so poor that it's Hobson's choice. They want to go somewhere else, paradoxically, because they are being denied their first choice – a high-quality, locally accessible service. Choice rhetoric has missed the one area where it has real meaning: for minority groups, for black and minority ethnic communities, for those socially excluded. Choice for them means recognition of difference, and redistribution to meet their needs in culturally appropriate ways. A choice of four or 40 hospitals is no choice at all if none tries to meet their cultural needs. Choice means empowering communities to design and run services relevant to their communities, to shape the local NHS or local authority to their cultural aspirations. Emphasising community engagement and social enterprise will achieve honest choice far more effectively.

bureaucracies and 'top-down managerialism'. To address this approach to healthcare he suggests three core principles for the public sector.

- The first principle is that the 'people' should be in control rather than top-down bureaucracies:

Local people should have the power to take the initiative, opening up services to mutual forms of ownership and engagement. Citizens should have more freedom to own, manage and direct public assets, from art galleries to local parks. There should also be clearer rights of redress. An NHS constitution would enshrine in statute the treatment to which every patient is entitled. The public should be empowered with high-quality, accessible performance data.

One may ask who the 'people' are? It has been suggested that the articulate affluent middle classes have been able to access and exercise choice in both education and health, and that those who need services more due to *social exclusion* are those least heard or 'empowered'. It is interesting to think how people may own, manage and direct health services.

- The second principle is that those who use services have responsibilities as well as rights:

    Where a service is abused, sanctions should prevail: those who miss an NHS appointment should pay a fine.

There may be an issue of social control here. Who is going to police this? Health professionals? Health service administrators? What would this potentially do to professional/public relationships for certain groups? Would nurses be able to stand apart from this process? Would health service employees be asked to intervene in a patient's inability to cooperate? Diamond uses the word 'abuse' when referring to service use. And on the surface it may seem self-evident that those who abuse should face sanctions. Another question that nurses should ask themselves is who defines what abuse is and who is going to deliver the sanctions?

- The third principle is to accept that there is a limit to what the State can do:

    Finally, genuine empowerment requires central government to modify its behaviour. [We] have to accept the limits of the traditional state as an instrument of social change.

Diamond's view demonstrates the thinking that underpins much public policy thinking: *We need a radical settlement for the next decade that passes back power, invests in public-service leadership, and rejects the post-1945 model of top-down change.*

It may be suggested that health professional groups and patients are two 'stakeholder' groups who have a say in how the NHS is run and how services are delivered. However, it has to be acknowledged that the government has introduced other powerful stakeholder groups, such as managers, who, in an increasingly budget-orientated era, may have other priorities. The role that professional groups play in this whole process is certainly under scrutiny and arguably (since the breakdown of the post-war consensus) is increasingly so.

O'Dowd (2007), in a report for the *British Medical Journal*, stated:

Clinicians should be consulted before any further NHS reforms are implemented, the former head of the NHS said last week. Sir Ian Carruthers, who was acting chief executive of the NHS for six months last year, has called for greater engagement with NHS staff on reforms in a report submitted to the Department of Health. Sir Ian, currently the chief executive of NHS South West, was commissioned by the government to carry out a review into the process of reconfiguration in the NHS and has reported back with several recommendations.

> *Involving clinicians and staff in developing proposals was critical, he concluded, and clinicians, staff, and their representatives needed to be more engaged in the process at a local, regional, and national level.*

This followed on from the Health Secretary's announcements that NHS changes would be continued, as Mayor (2006) reported:

> *The secretary of state for health in England, Patricia Hewitt, said that the traditional model of district general hospitals, which provide a range of care under one roof, was outdated. She argued that the next stage of development of the NHS was to put more power in the hands of patients and the local NHS.*
>
> *She confirmed that the great majority of hospitals would remain publicly owned, but they will be 'owned by the public rather than government', as NHS foundation trusts. She said that the NHS should use independent providers if they can provide better care and value for patients.*

In 2008, the then Prime Minister Gordon Brown announced in an open letter to NHS staff that the NHS would have a constitution outlining people's rights and responsibilities as citizens. That same letter discussed:

> *an NHS which is more personal and responsive to individual needs. Personalised not just because patients can get the treatment that they need when and where they want, but because from an early stage we are all given the information and advice to take greater responsibility for our own health.*

The debates concerning the future of the NHS may reflect the changing influences that professional groups have on healthcare delivery as much as they do the actual need for reform. Changing the way health is delivered may be challenging to those involved at the 'coal face'. Analysing arguments that are based on well-thought-out, reasoned and evidenced-based positions from those that are based on professional privilege and threat to professional autonomy is difficult. It is therefore important for professional groups to see beyond their own (narrow?) interests and engage in a policy debate that is clearly thought through and is explicit about whose interests are being served.

Activity 2.4   *Evidence-based practice and research*

- Use the internet to look at the Department of Health website, the websites of professional groups, and to search for specific terms.
- Is there any evidence that any professional group is feeling a challenge to its own perceived domain of influence and control?
- What is the PFI (Private Finance Initiative) and how is it affecting the provision of health services? In what way does it affect professionals' influence on this provision? Is there any evidence that it is eroding professional control?

A brief outline answer is given at the end of the chapter.

Historic milestones

The following dates are a little arbitrary but they do illustrate the rush of policy initiatives that are relevant for the NHS, particularly since the mid-1990s (see Day, 2006, ch. 2 and Barrett et al., 2005). The following indicate that even as far back as 1978 health policies indicate that 'working together' is a central idea in the delivery of healthcare. Indeed, the focus on this idea can be seen to be reinforced in many of the documents released since Alma-Ata.

1978

The World Health Organization (WHO) met at Alma-Ata and as a consequence the report *Health for All* was published. This is an important document as it sets out the philosophy for public health and primary care for member states (of which the UK is a signatory). It has to be recognised that this is non-binding agreement on countries, and as such could be seen more as a declaration of *intent* than an agreed action plan for which states would be held (publicly?) accountable.

There are two points to consider:

- IV. The people have the right and duty to participate individually and collectively in the planning and implementation of their healthcare.
- V. Governments have a responsibility for the health of their people that can be fulfilled only by the provision of adequate health and social measures.

This sets out clearly that people have a *right* to be involved and that it is a *legitimate government activity*. The latter point may seem obvious to a UK citizen born after the inception of the NHS, and indeed could be taken for granted that it is the State and the State only that provides this service. However, as policies develop, as private finances are brought to bear on the service, the assumption that it is the State only that is the key provider is being challenged with an increasing emphasis on the individual's own contribution to their health needs. The WHO declaration in addition to the rights of individuals also states they have *duties*. What may these be, how are they exercised and to what extent do individuals have the personal, social and financial resources to be able to fulfil their duties?

Activity 2.5 **Evidence-based practice and research**

- What is the World Health Organization?
- Where is it based?
- Who are its members?
- Who funds it?
- What are the ten key points that arise from the Alma-Ata declaration?

(Hint: See: www.who.int/en and *Primary Health Care: Report of the International Conference on Primary Health Care*, Alma-Ata, USSR, 6–12 September 1978.)

A brief outline answer is given at the end of the chapter.

An EU document *Partnerships for Health in Europe* states:

Mobilising different actors: partnerships for health
Putting health at the centre of EU-policy making is a shared responsibility. Different actors must work together if we are to succeed in achieving good health across the EU.

Citizens' health is to a great extent determined by individual choices on what people eat, smoke, drink and do. These choices are based on factors ranging from knowledge and information to socio-economic determinants. While Member

> *States are primarily responsible for promoting health and providing access to healthcare, citizens also have responsibility for promoting their own health.*
> (http://ec.europa.eu/health/ph_overview/
> Documents/partnerships_health_en.pdf, p5)

This statement clearly sets out the role of citizens in their own health. The challenge for nurses is working with people to understand this responsibility and helping people to develop skills to exercise this responsibility. For example, if there is a lack of knowledge about healthy eating, what is the nurse's role in increasing this knowledge to allow people to make better choices about food?

1979

The election of Margaret Thatcher (Conservative), who sought to challenge State and professional intervention in public services, paradoxically increased State control in some areas such as local government. The scope of Thatcher's reforms of the public sector is too vast to be covered here, but it includes such events as the 1984 miners' strike which established the government's power to decide economic and energy policy by effectively breaking the power of the National Union of Miners and, by implication, of trade unions generally. It has a resonance for the professions in that this signalled the intent that no vested interests should take precedence in deciding public policy.

Many nurses, historically, have situated themselves outside these arguments by having a no-strike policy based in an organisation that could be seen by outsiders as a 'trade union' that goes under the name of a 'Royal College'. In addition to its education and health policy roles, the Royal College of Nursing (RCN) has a remit to look after the pay and conditions of nurses. The RCN is also a fully constituted union, a registered charity and a professional organisation. However, it could be argued that there is a an inherent contradiction in the work of the College in that on one hand it seeks objectively to contribute to health policy issues, while on the other having the interest of nurses as health service employees. As the NHS changes the skill mix of its employees (taking on more assistant practitioners and less registered nurses), this will pose a challenge to nurses within the RCN as well as outside. Is there a public interest issue here? Is it a more appropriate and cheaper (?) skill mix that will clash with the registered nurses' needs and wishes to be employed in more numbers? Thatcher may have won the argument in 1984 but the issue remains: vested professional interests (more registered nurses) v. public interests (a cheaper more appropriate workforce). Of course, this can be seen as a false choice, but professionals have to research and argue why their case serves the public and is not a self-serving policy.

1989

The Department of Health (DH, 1989a) published principles that required health and social care services to collaborate in order to be jointly financially responsible for the provision of care in the community, with an emphasis on *effective joint working*. In the same year the NHS faced major structural change in that the 'internal market' was introduced. *Purchasers* (health authorities and some GPs) bought services from *Providers* (acute hospitals, ambulance services etc). Providers became independently managed Trusts in a quasi-competitive market. The White Paper, *Working for Patients* (DH, 1989b), emphasised making the health service more responsive to patient need and to allow money to treat patients to cross administrative boundaries, thus laying the ground for interprofessional working.

The concept of a 'seamless service' is emphasised in a further range of government documents. A seamless service means providing care across organisational boundaries and needs teamworking between professional groups (DH, 1996a, b; NHS Executive, 1996). In the field of mental health, health authorities were to work with a range of other agencies to provide care for people (DH, 1998a).

1997

Tony Blair's 'New Labour' government was elected in May 1997 and the White Paper, *The New NHS – Modern, Dependable* (DH, 1997), was an attempt to turn the NHS into a more *modern* organisation – 'modernisation' was to become a key idea in the public services. The idea was to encourage the integration of care through partnerships by agencies and organisations. Professional and organisational boundaries should not hinder people from getting the care they required while the NHS would seek to work more closely with services responsible for housing, education and social care. People should be seen to be at the centre of things rather than as passive recipients. Day (2006) argues that three main themes emerge from this White Paper:

- partnership working;
- patient-centred care;
- organisational changes to make these possible.

These themes were part of New Labour's attempt at getting 'joined up thinking' in the public sector, which resulted in the setting up of *Health Action Zones* (DH, 1998b), whereby all professionals involved in health should get together to plan and deliver services.

1998

The White Paper, *A First-class Service: Quality in the new NHS* (DH, 1998c), paved the way for national service frameworks (NSFs), which again places emphasis on partnership working. This involves cross-agency and sector working (primary care, community care and hospitals) as well as professional groups. For example, the NSF for Older People suggests a single assessment process to overcome the need for each single health and social care professional to undertake their separate assessments.

1999

Another key document is *Making a Difference* (DH, 1999), targeting nurses, midwives and health visitors to engage in 'working with others':

> *Effective care and treatment are the product of team effort. Seamless services demand interagency working and collaboration. Subject to proper regard for public protection, there is no place for rigid demarcation of role boundaries in a modern service. As services develop, local action is needed to help multi-disciplinary and interagency teams work effectively. The challenge is as much for colleagues in other disciplines as it is for nurses, midwives and health visitors. But nurses, midwives and health visitors are well placed to help foster team work with other health and social care professionals.*
>
> (p70)

Activity 2.6   *Critical thinking*

Note the phrase *no place for rigid demarcation of role boundaries* in the above *Making a Difference* document. What does this mean and why do you think it was necessary to write this? Think about the roles that junior doctors, staff nurses and care assistants carry out. Is there an overlap? Are roles changing? Can you identify tasks that one professional carries out that could be done by another worker?

A brief outline answer is given at the end of the chapter.

2000

The NHS Plan: A plan for investment a plan for reform (DH, 2000a) follows up on the previous White Paper, *The New NHS – Modern, Dependable*. It sets out a strategy to modernise the NHS and to address some of its shortcomings, notably role demarcation and professional boundaries. In line with *Making a Difference*, nurses were to expand roles, which has implications for the relationship between them and the medical profession. An example is the nurse practitioner in a minor injury unit who sees patients who would otherwise have been seen by doctors. He or she may undertake a consultation (often using a method followed by medical practitioners), make diagnoses of minor injury or illness, initiate investigations or treatments and devise management plans, including follow-up. The education of such practitioners often involves the medical profession. It may be noted that doctors have always been involved in nursing education but now there may be a real difference in what that education entails. The focus now may be on the sharing of what was traditionally medical skills and knowledge (including history-taking) for clinical practice rather than on teaching about diseases or anatomy and physiology.

Activity 2.7   *Evidence-based practice and research*

Traditionally, nurses and doctors have either 'admitted' (nurses) or 'clerked' (house officers) patients, or they have 'assessed' or 'undertaken a consultation' often quite separately. In hospital the same admission process had usually resulted in two visits to the same patient by a nurse and a doctor. In primary care a patient used to see a doctor or a practice nurse for two quite different reasons.

- Enquire of a nurse the difference between 'admission or nursing assessment' and medical 'clerking'. Enquire of a doctor what 'clerking' entails.
- Enquire in a primary care setting, e.g. a GP practice, or minor injury unit, what 'history-taking' or a 'medical consultation' means.
- Note the differences and the similarities between the approaches. Is this evidence of professional overlap?

As the questions depend on your own findings, there is no outline answer at the end of the chapter.

Barrett et al. (2005) state that *the European Union has placed an emphasis on a right of parity for health and social care . . . in member states locating responsibility for the organisation of care with policy makers answerable to the general public* (p11). The EU provides a framework for health policy and has published a European Community Health Strategy 2000 (European Commission, 2000), which intended to *set up a new mechanism, the* **European Health Forum**, *to give the public health community at large an opportunity to play a role in the development of health policy.* The reference to the *public health community* may include professionals in health and public services, but does not necessarily mean the general public. If, however, the public health community (doctors, nurses, researchers, health service managers) involve the wider population in discussions of health needs and priorities this may be a step towards making *policy makers answerable to the public.*

Therefore, it may be argued that at an international level there is a 'surface' coherence in stated health policy between the national UK government and the wider pan-national World Health Organization (1978, Alma-Ata) and the EU. This coherence is on the issue of public involvement in health services. At a deeper level, the detail of what this means in each individual member state, each individual health service and for the professional groups within each health service will be different. 'Public involvement' as a concept needs further exploration . . . how UK nurses help the public to be involved also will require much further examination by the nursing profession itself as well as other stakeholders.

2003

The Commission for Patient and Public Involvement in Health (CPPIH) was set up in January 2003. It was an independent, non-departmental public body, sponsored by the Department of Health.

CPPIH's role was to make sure the public is involved in decision making about health and health services in England. There are over 400 Patient and Public Involvement (PPI) Forums, one for each NHS Trust in England, and they work to ensure that local people and communities have a say in improving local health services.

PPI Forums are made up of groups of volunteers in local communities who are enthusiastic about helping patients and members of the public to influence the way that local healthcare is delivered. Forum members come from a broad variety of backgrounds and have a range of experiences and skills.

CPPIH was responsible for submitting reports to and advising the government on how the PPI system is functioning. It liaises with national bodies such as the now defunct Healthcare Commission on patient and public involvement issues, and makes recommendations to these bodies and the Department of Health as appropriate.

CPPIH gathered information and opinion from PPI Forums, channelled through its shared information system in order to ensure that the bodies it reports to are acting upon patients' and the public's views.

2004

The NHS Improvement Plan: Putting people at the heart of public services (DH, 2004) reaffirms the concept of modernising the NHS to be responsive to people's needs. The document argues:

> *The next stage in the NHS's journey is to ensure that a drive for responsive, convenient and personalised services takes root across the whole of the NHS and for all patients.*
> (DH, 2004, Executive Summary, section 1)

> *A much wider choice of different types of health services will become available to NHS patients, to enable personalised care, faster treatment, personal support for people with long-term conditions and better social care.*
> (DH, 2004, Executive Summary, section 3)

And . . .

> *NHS patients will also be able to choose from a growing range of independent providers, with their diagnosis and treatment paid for by the NHS. To support capacity and choice, by 2008, independent sector providers will provide up to 15% of procedures on behalf of the NHS.*
> (DH, 2004, Executive Summary, section 3)

Note how *choice* and the use of the *independent (private) sector* are again central to the modernisation agenda.

CASE STUDY: CPPHI SURVEY, MARCH 2007

The following was published on the now defunct CPPHI website:

PATIENT FORUMS SAY 'STOP THE MIXED-SEX WARD SHAME'

Patient Forums have welcomed the report from the Chief Nursing Officer, Professor Christine Beasley, into the greater need for single-sex hospital wards. Following their own in-depth research into the experience of over 2,500 patients in March (2007), Patient Forums highlighted the continuing unacceptable level of patients who still have to share wards with members of the opposite sex – causing them needless concern and anxiety. This is exacerbated by patients who were forced to share mixed-sex toilet facilities, leaving many feeling awkward and embarrassed.

Figures from the Patient Forum's 'Care Watch' survey, which was conducted throughout 95 Acute and Mental Health NHS Trusts across England, showed that:

- in Acute Trusts, *25 per cent* of patients had to share a ward/bay with members of the opposite sex;
- in these cases, *62 per cent* were only separated by a screen;
- however, over a third of those surveyed (*37 per cent*) were not happy sharing a ward/bay with members of the opposite sex;
- in Acute Trusts, a quarter of patients (*25 per cent*) did not have access to single sex toilet facilities within easy reach.

Speaking on behalf of the Oxford Radcliffe Hospitals PPI Forum, Chair Jacquie Pearce-Gervis said:

Naturally, we welcome this report which will give hospital trusts advice on how to improve their single sex wards.

Patient Forum members heard many anecdotes from patients who felt ill-at-ease or in some cases unsafe sleeping in a mixed ward, or they asked to be moved to a single sex ward, when one became available.

Many patients are concerned that their stay in hospital will be made uncomfortable by having to share their ward with members of the opposite sex. Patients said they would not stay on a mixed sex ward if it was of their own choosing; having said that, they realised that in cases of emergencies, this was not always possible.

While improvements are needed, we would like to see an eradication of mixed sex wards in order for all patients to spend their time in hospital recovering and not worrying that their dignity or privacy could be compromised.

Source: Commission for Patient and Public Involvement in Health (2007).

The view from a PPI member (anonymised), December 2007 (before LINk implementation)

Because we did this (the 'Care Watch' survey) as part of a national survey by our commission (the CPPIH) we sent it to them so as to form part of

---

CASE STUDY continued

an overall picture of where the NHS was going on this subject. The commission publish their overall figures and send it to the DOH. For our part we send our figures to the hospital trust board as we are required to do as it is a formal inspection.

Three of us sit on the PEAT (patient environment action team) committee at the hospital where things like this are discussed with members of the trust board, other managers, matrons etc. It meets every month. Every three months we do another inspection with managers of various departments. We would normally do a routine follow-up inspection but I doubt whether we will be able to get this done before the end of PPIs as we have to square up all our other work to be able to hand over to LINks. It seems that we have come out fairly well out of the survey.

I am on the select committee that will appoint a Host for the (local) LINk. The Host will be an arm's length body between the city council and the LINk. I still remain to be convinced about the change to LINks and at this stage I am not too sure of the benefits of it.

I do however know that although it was a tough battle at first that we have got through a lot of good work in the PPI forum and it was not just paying lip service. We do have many instances of where we have managed to change the opinions of the trust board by working with them. We now have situations where they come to us to ask us for our opinions instead of us having to go to them.

Activity 2.8   *Evidence-based practice and research*

This activity involves the Patient Advice and Liaison Services (PALS) and Patient and Public Involvement (PPI) Forums. Go to the Department of Health website (www.dh.gov.uk/), click on 'Policy and Guidance' and then look for 'Patient and Public Involvement' for the outline of how the NHS had been asked to implement this aspect of a government initiative. Follow the link to Patient Advice and Liaison Services and look at 'Key messages for NHS organisations: the national evaluation of PALS'. An extract is shown below.

What points would be applicable in your immediate experience? Produce an example from your practice, such as powerful individual stories from patients. Can you give an example of how and where this has impacted on practice in your locality? Can you uncover how PALS has 'enhanced the patient experience'? Give a concrete example.

As the example will be based on your own experience, there is no outline answer at the end of the chapter.

PALS

- PALS can contribute to enhancing the patient experience and improving services, helping your organisation be fit for purpose and meet the requirements of regulatory bodies such as the Healthcare Commission.
- The characteristics of successful PALS include:
  - a history of support for PPI in the organisation together with Board-level support for PALS;
  - a senior manager with change management skills, giving strategic leadership to PALS;
  - integration with PPI, partnerships, clinical governance and risk management;
  - good information systems for sharing and integrating PALS intelligence across the organisation;
  - engagement with Trust/PCT staff;
  - networking across the health community.
- PALS can often tell very powerful individual stories about the positive impact of their services for users.
- PALS actively filter potential complaints and ensure that issues that are brought to the Trusts are cogent and appropriate.
- Where Trusts and PCTs have well-resourced and supported PALS, they play an important role in improving the patient experience and supporting service improvement.
- Where Trusts and PCTs give PALS very little resource or support, they get very little in the way of activity or impact.

2006

In August 2005 the Department of Health reviewed patient and public involvement in the provision of health services. Following this review, in January 2006 the White Paper, *Our Health, Our Say, Our Care: A new direction for community services*, was published. This set out to promote further patient *independence, choice and control*, building on earlier patient involvement philosophies. Following on from this in the White Paper, *A Stronger Local Voice*, the DH (2006) argues:

> The purpose of the new framework is to make sure that the needs, preferences and involvement of local people, including those that are seldom heard, are central to the planning, development and delivery of health and social care services.

This has led to the government's proposed legislation 'Local Government and Public Involvement in Health' bill which set up 150 Local Involvement Networks (LINks) to replace the 400 Public Forums and the Commission for Patient and Public Involvement in Health (CPPIH).

Local Involvement Networks

In April 2008, Local Involvement Networks (LINks) replaced Patient Forums. The DH (2007b) argues that *LINks are being introduced to help strengthen the system that enables communities to influence the care they receive.*
Backed up by certain powers, LINks:

- *provide everyone in the community – from individuals to voluntary groups – with the chance to say what they think about local health and social care services – what is working and what is not;*

- *give people the chance to influence how services are planned and run;*
- *feedback to services what people have said about services so that things can be improved.*

(DH, 2007b)

However, prior to the setting up of LINks there were concerns expressed about their scope and their ability to fund activities that will truly support public involvement. Thus:

Patients' voice slips away quietly?

Sharon Grant, Chair of CPPIH, voices her concerns about legislation, which has its second reading in Parliament this week, that changes to the way the public can influence the NHS:

> *Slipping through Parliament this week, will be legislation which once again will alter drastically the way in which patients and the public can influence the public service they most value – the NHS.*

> *Woven into a local government Bill, without a Health Minister in sight, 12 clauses will abolish the Commission for Patient and Public Involvement, established only in 2003. Also abolished will be the 400 or so independent Patient and Public Involvement Forums, which it supports. They have some 5,000 volunteer members across the country, and are themselves just a little more than three years old.*

(CPPIH, January 2007)

And:

Public will walk away from health's 'weakest LINk'

The CPPIH welcomes today's thorough report from the Health Select Committee into Patient and Public Involvement in the NHS.

Sharon Grant, Chair of the Commission for Patient and Public Involvement in Health commented:

> *We concur with its substantial conclusion that the current proposals to reform the system for public voice in health are flawed.*

> *In particular the lack of clarity about the new LINks role and structure is a real cause for concern. If after detailed examination, senior MP's could not make sense of the Government's proposals, then there must be a real question mark over whether the public will be able to make use of it.*

(CPPIH, April 2007)

Whether this is a case of special pleading from a vested interest or is borne out in reality will need studying. It does illustrate that when it comes to public policy there are disagreements about implementation if not always about the goals. Thus public bodies, government departments, the public themselves as well as professionals may agree that 'involvement' (insert your own idea here) is 'a good thing', but how the idea gets put into practice highlights differences in the way groups of people see how to implement their arguments over funding the action or concerns over their own role (after all, if a role is to disappear, especially one funded by government, it is natural that staff may feel threatened – regardless of whether the threat is real or imaginary).

Activity 2.9   *Critical thinking*

We are left with four key questions about patient involvement. How do you think you would answer the following?

1. What are the different approaches used to encourage 'user involvement'? What are the different methods used to access user views?
2. What exactly does 'involvement' mean? Does this mean the individual's involvement in his or her own care decisions on a one-to-one basis with a professional; involvement in decisions at their community level (for example, their own GP practice or as a patient in the ward setting) or involvement at more strategic level – Hospital or Primary Care Trust, or even at the Strategic Health Authority level?
3. Have you observed an NHS organisation, such as your placement, engaging with patient involvement?
4. Have you observed any evidence of user involvement making a difference in your placement?

Do you have any suggestions about how user involvement might make a difference in your placement? Discuss your ideas with your mentor.

An outline answer is given at the end of the chapter.

Since the introduction of LINks, the government has emphasised the idea of the public's engagement in healthcare delivery. This may, of course, relate to the idea of people as active citizens with rights and responsibilities. The Department of Health, for example, has published documents on 'experience' and 'engagement' – that is to say, there is a focus on the public being fully involved in the NHS and not just as passive consumers of health services.

In 2008 the government commissioned a review of 'customer experience', followed by the concept of patient and public engagement (PPE), for example as highlighted in a document called *The Engagement Cycle* (DH, 2009a), which discusses patients' engagement in commissioning services (buying healthcare services). Another initiative is a focus on gathering feedback from patients outlined in *Understanding What Matters: A guide to using patient feedback to transform care* (DH, 2009b). In fact, 2009 was a busy year for even more DH guidance, such as *Putting Patients at the Heart of Care* (DH, 2009c) and *Helping the NHS Put Patients at the Heart of Care* (DH, 2009d).

In April 2010 legislation came into force (DH, 2009e) that will require NHS organisations (for example, primary care trusts) to explain how they have acted on patient and public feedback. These obligations will have legal backing.

Under the concept of PPE then, the DH has asked (and legally requires) NHS organisations and staff to engage more fully and respond to the public. Whether the public perceives engagement at the level discussed in DH publications is a matter for reflection.

2007 NHS reconfiguration

The NHS throughout its history has been under constant scrutiny and subject to major changes or 'reforms'. It is undergoing further changes to the way it works called *reconfiguration*. In October 2006, Sir Ian Carruthers was commissioned to review how the changing NHS is structured and how it deals with improving its services. He argued, emphasising involvement by key stakeholders:

Change can all too frequently lead to a loss of public confidence in service providers if the process is not managed carefully, and stakeholders are not fully engaged as early as possible.

(DH, 2007a)

One of the main recommendations in the review is:

Clinical and staff involvement in developing proposals is critical; we need greater engagement of clinicians, staff and their representatives in the process at a local, regional and national level.

(DH, 2007a)

Thus, this is a continuation of the idea that NHS services, as they change, must involve a wide range of people and not just the professionals or managers alone. However, what needs to be examined is how this should be put into action.

A key question for nurses might be: 'In what way exactly are patients and clinical nursing staff engaged, involved, consulted in the whole process of NHS change?'

Patricia Hewitt, then Secretary of State for Health, discussed the impact of reconfiguration thus:

*The Government . . . will move towards a health service focused on **prevention** as much as cure, and increasingly **shift away from hospital care** to community based services. As we do this, the NHS has a historic opportunity to become an agent for regeneration and renewal. In many areas, the NHS is the major local employer and a major customer for local suppliers. Decisions about the location of buildings, equipment and services, can be a major contributor towards the regeneration of deprived neighbourhoods.*

Therefore, I will be insisting that from now on the NHS takes account of the impact of reconfiguration of services on the local economy and local communities. We will be reviewing our guidance to the NHS to ensure that when a new hospital or health centre is proposed, a key factor in the decision making process will be the benefit to the local community in terms of creating employment, buying goods from local suppliers, designing new buildings that save energy and are pleasant places to work and visit, and providing sustainable transport policies.

(Speech to the UK Public Health Associations annual forum in Telford, 2007 – see www.dh.gov.uk media centre)

All of this may seem far removed from the everyday work of the registered nurse. However, what we need to note is the drive towards fundamental changes in how and where staff and patients receive and deliver healthcare. Key ideas are *prevention* as well as *cure*, *community* as well as *hospital*-based care. Therefore, nurses will have to respond to these policy initiatives and understand that it may be the case that some clinical units close and other provision may come into place. This illustrates the political nature of health service delivery and the need for health service staff to respond creatively and critically, with patients, to the new pressures.

This *public health orientation* to the NHS is not new. However, it does mean a cultural shift for many professional staff in the way they have traditionally understood the priorities for health services. The public have shown that major changes (such as possible closures to Accident and Emergency (A & E) departments) will not go through without protest. While the government may suggest a shift to the community and hence a logical need to change how services are provided, people in the UK are not letting this go unchallenged. In London it was reported that nine A & E departments could be closed in a reconfiguration of services elsewhere (BBC, 2006b). This, of course, provoked much concern.

Our NHS, Our Future, *2007*

The Department of Health had another initiative which states:

> Our NHS, Our Future *is a wide-ranging review (led by Lord Darzi) to identify the way forward for the NHS over the next decade and beyond. It is vital that local staff, who are best placed to know how to meet patients' needs, are at the centre of the debate.*

The review attempted to engage the public in the discussion, generating online surveys and a website to encourage feedback (www.nhs.uk/ournhs). During 2007, there were a number of 'engagement events' generating a report, such as the '18 September 2007 Nationwide Consultative Event' (DH, 2007c). The report, by research company Opinion Leader, is an in-depth analysis of the views of over 1,000 patients, members of the public, and health and social care staff.

> *Results from the day showed that people are generally quite satisfied with the Health Service – and continue to support a tax funded NHS. The majority of people are very supportive of NHS staff and the work they do, but believe a change in focus from caring for people once they are ill, to preventing illness should be taken in the future. Access to local, out of hours GPs, and worries about hospital cleanliness were at the top of most people's concerns.*

(DH, 2007c)

Activity 2.10 *Critical thinking*

1. Sitzia et al. (2006) report a small research study involving interviewing 59 cancer service users and NHS staff to evaluate the Cancer Partnership Project (CPP). The CPP, they state, is a leading Patient and Public Involvement (PPI) policy. The focus should be on service improvement involving service users and NHS staff. The results of the interviews, they argue, demonstrate that these partnership groups may be useful but difficulties and complexities remain as part of meaningful 'cultural change'.

- This is one study – to what extent can it be generalised to the wider UK context?
- What might the authors imply by 'meaningful cultural change' – from what to what?

2. Elston and Holloway (2001) interviewed General Practitioners (GPs), nurses and practice managers in three Primary Care centres to compare their perspectives on changes to primary care, including moves towards interprofessional collaboration and the development of their professional roles. They identified that *professional identities* and *traditional power structures* generated conflict. They concluded, *it will take a new generation of health professionals to bring about an interprofessional culture in the NHS* (p 19).

- How do the findings of this study relate to Sitzia et al.'s ? Are there any concepts in common? Professional identity, culture and traditional power structures will be addressed in more detail in later chapters.

A brief outline answer is given at the end of the chapter.

The Care Quality Commission, 2008

Health and social care services are subject to external inspection in addition to the guidance and policy set out by the DH. Therefore, staff will be subject to policies and practices that have a direct impact on their work. The Health and Social Care Act 2008 established a single, integrated regulator for health and adult social care – the Care Quality Commission (CQC) – to replace previous monitoring and inspection bodies. In July 2009 the CQC launched 'Voices into Action' – an initiative that accords with the DH's emphasis on PPE. The CQC (2009) states:

> We want you to have a bigger say in how the health and social care services that you use should be improved. Our new Voices into Action statement says that we will: involve the people who use care services in everything we do and ensure that care services respond to what people tell them.

This will be achieved by the use of surveys, consultations and the LINks. Therefore, this appears to be a reinforcement of the idea that patients and clients of healthcare services are again to be seen as active participants whose views must be taken into account by all staff.

The impact of technology

Technology changes human behaviour. There is much written about how technology and its use affect human culture (Marshall McLuhan: *we shape our tools and they in turn shape us*) and the way we then behave towards each other. The development of new techniques and the availability of machines, drugs and information processes do not act in a neutral way upon those who use and develop them.

An easy example is to think of how our lives have been changed by the mobile phone or the internet. Once seen as an innovation (and an expensive one at that, only for the use of City of London financiers), the mobile phone has now become every teenager's toy. Text messaging exploded in use in a completely unforeseen way. It may be interesting to think for a few moments that, if mobile phones were taken away from, say, the under 25-year-olds, a revolt would possibly follow – a revolt that would be secondary in size and ferocity only to the revolt by the older generations if the motor car were suddenly banned. The point is that technology in many cases irreversibly changes the way we go about our daily living. We make choices based on the availability and use of technology until, in some cases, we become dependent on it.

Technology can mean the development of new drugs, surgical techniques and equipment for invasive (i.e. penetrating body tissue – tubes inserted into major blood vessels to measure blood pressure in the heart) and non-invasive (such as pulse oximeters) physiological monitoring machines.

Technology also means communications technology. Apply this to healthcare. How has the advance of technology impacted on nursing care? Email, video conferencing, telemedicine, electronic patient records, all have the potential to enhance inter-professional collaboration and communication, irrespective of geography. Patients are becoming more used to finding help and assistance using the internet. How does this impact on the way patients now talk about their health with GPs and other health professionals?

The next generation of web technologies are allowing discussion, creativity and interaction rather than being just information sources (Boulos and Wheeler, 2007). Will we see patient support groups using web technologies to discuss all aspects of their care? How, for example, will patients and clients discuss treatment options or care experiences using this technology? Does this mean that healthcare staff will have to become more knowledgeable about the use of such technologies in the need to more fully engage with the changing demands made by patients? See the Case Study below.

CASE STUDY: TELEMEDICINE – EVOLUTION OR EXTINCTION?

New technologies open up opportunities to work with others in ways that may not have been possible before. Telemedicine could be seen to be just such a tool that not only improves care but changes the nature of working relationships. Telemedicine is used to refer to any application of information and communications technology which removes or reduces the effect of distance between healthcare settings. It has been argued that telemedicine will have a significant effect on the way that clinical care is delivered in the future (Scottish Telemedicine Initiative, 2000). For example, consultants in A & E departments, if linked with a minor injury unit situated some distance away, could view X-rays, or the actual patient, thus enabling and supporting nurse (or emergency care) practitioners to make decisions about the need to admit or treat certain patient cases.

However, as with many initiatives, things do not always go to plan. Just as the explosion in predictive text messaging was discovered as a happy accident by mobile phone companies, so technologies have lives (and deaths) of their own.

Despite high expectations, telemedicine (and telehealthcare) systems, which enable doctors to interact with patients many miles away via video, digital imaging and electronic data transmission, have had only limited impact on the National Health Service, according to a study sponsored by the ESRC.

The expected revolution in medicine, overcoming problems of access to specialist care and speeding up referrals and diagnosis, has simply not happened, say researchers led by Professor Carl May, of the University of Newcastle upon Tyne.

'Telemedicine' is disappearing, in stark contrast to the apparent success of telephone services on which clinical staff decide the urgency of patients' injuries or illnesses, and advice lines such as NHS Direct.

Resistance from professionals is often blamed, but the real reason is often a failure to think through the organisational problems involved in integrating new technology into everyday NHS activity.

Telemedicine lets doctors deal remotely with patients over a live video-conferencing link where a face-to-face consultation may be difficult or time-wasting, such as when patients live in isolated rural areas. And it makes it easier to share pictures and data with experts in different parts of the UK or, potentially, other countries.

But while 'telemedicine' is on the wane, new portable 'telecare' systems for monitoring people with illnesses such as diabetes, asthma, and respiratory and cardiovascular disorders, are under development.

These new systems connect patients with the NHS using mobile or fixed phones to send data about health problems, enabling early intervention when needed, and potentially reducing hospital admissions. But they face

---

CASE STUDY *continued*

> *similar problems of integration in a health service which is not a single organisation, but rather a federation of more than 700 NHS trusts, each with its own procurement and management structure.*
>
> (ESRC, 2005)

Knowledge about health and illness is becoming more easily accessible and this will change the role of health professionals in relation to the demands made by users. The lesson here is that technological change is inevitable and widespread, and changes the nature of human interaction and relationships. However, predicting that change and responding to it is far more of a challenge.

Poor collaborative practice

Several cases have highlighted that professions and agencies have not always been working well together. The result has been very serious for some. Children's services exemplify some of the issues.

Children have probably been abused and killed as long as there has been human history. Each death is tragic and not all are the result of poor agency working. However, poor communication (and training) between professions and agencies may have been implicated in the following:

- Dennis O'Neill, 1945;
- Maria Colwell, 1973;
- Jasmine Beckford, 1984;
- Heidi Koseda, 1984;
- Tyra Henry, 1984;
- Kimberley Carlile, 1986;
- Doreen Mason, 1987;
- Leanne White, 1992;
- Riki Neave, 1994;
- Chelsea Brown, 1999;
- Lauren Wright, 2000;
- Victoria Climbié, 2000;
- Ainlee Labonte, 2002;
- Baby Peter, 2008.

The Monkton Report (1948) into the death of Dennis O'Neill (a twelve-year-old boy killed by his foster father) noted:

- confusion between the two local authorities looking after him;
- conflicting reports on the boy's well-being by childcare staff;
- staff shortages;
- miscommunication.

Maria Colwell (1973) was seven years old and died in Brighton after being starved and beaten by her stepfather. An inquiry by the Department of Health found there were

50 official visits to the family, including from social workers, health visitors, police and housing officers. All agencies involved in the case were criticised.

Ainlee Labonte (2002) was two years old and was starved and tortured to death by her parents. An inquiry into her death found that the health and social workers who should have protected her did not do so because they were paralysed with fear of her parents. It criticised the staff and agencies involved for poor communication and for failing to carry out a proper assessment of the risks faced by Ainlee.

Following the death of Victoria Climbié (abused and tortured by her aunt and the man she lived with), the government published *Every Child Matters* (DCSF, 2003). There was also a formal response to the report into her death, which preceded this document.

Every Child Matters emphasised four key themes in order to build on existing plans to strengthen preventative services.

- Increasing the focus on supporting families and carers.
- Ensuring necessary intervention takes place before children reach crisis point and protecting children from falling through the net.
- Addressing the underlying problems identified in the report into the death of Victoria Climbié – *weak accountability* and *poor integration* (our emphasis).
- Ensuring that the people working with children are valued, rewarded and trained.

The death of 'Baby Peter' in August 2007, in the same London borough as Victoria Climbié, highlighted the need for robust child protection policies. The government had published *Every Child Matters: The next steps* (DCSF, 2004), and had passed the Children Act 2004, providing a legal framework for developing more effective and accessible services focused around the needs of children, young people and families.

For a more detailed discussion of these cases, see Batty (2003).

In addition to child abuse there have been other high-profile examples of professional 'failure and abuse', e.g. deaths could have been prevented with better training, communication and monitoring systems.

- **Beverly Allitt** was a registered nurse who murdered children. The resulting enquiry showed issues around communication between agencies that may have prevented her from working with children.
- **Bristol Royal Infirmary** children's heart surgery inquiry was:

   an account of people who cared greatly about human suffering, and were dedicated and well-motivated. Sadly, some lacked insight and their behaviour was flawed. Many failed to communicate with each other, and to work together effectively for the interests of their patients. There was a lack of leadership, and of teamwork.

   (www.bristol-inquiry.org.uk)

- **Harold Shipman**, a GP in Hyde, Manchester, who was convicted of the murder of 15 of his patients in 2000.
  The Shipman Inquiry (2005) noted that he was responsible for 215 deaths and that:

   [t]he majority of those deaths were followed by cremation. Before a cremation can be authorised, a second doctor must confirm the cause of death and the cremation documentation must be checked by a third doctor employed at the crematorium. These procedures are intended to provide a safeguard for the public against concealment of homicide. Yet, even with these procedures in place, Shipman was able to kill 215 people without detection.

The inquiry thus found systems failures in that, despite having a drugs conviction, Shipman was still able to stockpile controlled drugs, he was able to bypass the normal coroner's investigations and that his activities went unchecked by other fellow professionals for many years. This case has implications for the regulation of medical practitioners and for the systems that are in place that should provide checks and balances for the professionals involved. It can be seen to be another issue that challenges the lone professional worker isolated from wider scrutiny, support, training and monitoring. It may also challenge the idea of professional self-regulation.

Miller (2004) argued:

> Organisational and professional partiality and territoriality, with their inherent tendencies towards restrictive practices alongside organisational philosophical and cultural differences, have long been a detriment to the service user and have contributed to policy failure.

(p132)

This is an attack on old-style practices, whereby professionals stay within their own 'comfort zones', failing to communicate or even understanding each other's roles. It seems to say that people's needs can then fall between two stools. One reason this occurred may have been down to how professionals are educated.

D'Amour et al. (2005) argue that, as professional groups are educated separately, they are socialised into 'discipline-specific thinking'. This affects the way they work with their patient groups and the way they go about delivering a service. If we think of nursing as a discipline, for example, this suggests that nurses are developing their own theory and their own methods of practice, which do not open themselves up to other ways of 'non-nursing' thinking or practising.

So, for example, nurses have explicitly used concepts such as the 'nursing process' based on nursing models (e.g. the Roper, Logan and Tierney Activities of Daily Living model), which have a particular way of seeing the needs of patients and what nursing work is all about. Put very simply, nursing work understands that the patient has spiritual, moral, psychological and social needs as well as biological needs. Nursing may be about helping the individual to undertake everyday activities overcoming illness as well as maintaining health.

The traditional contrast is with medical ways of thinking. Again, very simply (and to do an injustice to many doctors) medicine focuses on the biology, putting right problems with human physiology and anatomy, curing illness and disease, or managing pain and death. So, nurses are deemed to 'care' while doctors 'cure'.

Interprofessional education and collaboration should be about challenging some of these base assumptions on both sides of the professional divide. Interprofessional education will be discussed in more detail in Chapter 7.

As nursing begins to adopt new roles and new ways of thinking, the paradox is that collaboration results not because of any shared understanding but because nurses are taking on medical tasks and beginning to look, talk and act like doctors. Do you think the nurses in the Case Study below are 'caring'?

The recognition that old ways of working have not served people well and the development of new and expanded roles in the NHS are pushing healthcare groups into a rethink of their proper place and how they ought to work together in the future.

CASE STUDY: THE CHANGING ROLE OF NURSE PRACTITIONERS IN THE UK

Interprofessional working can be seen in practice in the UK, in various schemes run by Morecambe Bay NHS Trust. The Trust serves people living in urban and rural areas in parts of Cumbria, Lancashire and north Yorkshire. In response to the legal requirements to cut junior doctors' hours, nurses are being trained to take on new roles. Two nurses – a theatre sister and a ward sister – were being trained in an 18-month project (due to finish in November 2004) to become colorectal surgical assistants. Training includes opening and closing surgical wounds. The Trust has also taken on Swiss nurses, who perform some anaesthetic work in Switzerland, to see if this role could be usefully implemented in the UK.

Concern has been expressed as to how this new trend will be received by doctors, but it is believed that these types of pilot programme will provide an opportunity for different and 'smarter' ways of working.'

Sources: Rayner (2003); BMA (2005).

Collaborating with others in a rural environment

Healthcare delivery in a rural setting brings its own challenges. The relative lack of public transport, rural deprivation, loss of services and increasingly elderly populations added to family, social and geographical mobility, means that services and those who provide them are faced with different issues from those faced in metropolitan districts. Added to distances and centralisation of some services (see the Case Study below) and a reduction in GP cover, health professionals have to respond to provide a comprehensive service which means working in new ways.

CASE STUDY: RURALITY AND HEALTHCARE – CANCER SERVICES

Research suggests that there are rural–urban differences in health outcomes, and the belief that rural patients have a health advantage over their urban counterparts may be incorrect (Campbell et al., 2000). In response, different approaches to healthcare provision may need to be taken in rural and urban areas, as often those that work well in urban areas do not translate to a rural situation. This may increase the need for closer collaboration and 'cross boundary working', i.e. one professional group undertaking the work traditionally done by another (e.g. non-medical prescribers).

Recognition of the benefits of specialised cancer care, for example, has led to the reshaping of cancer services in the UK. This has resulted in a move towards centralisation, which has implications for those living in rural areas (Campbell et al., 2001). This study investigated whether survival from cancer differed for patients resident in a rural and an urban area. It was found that patient distance from the nearest cancer centre can affect cancer survival (Campbell et al., 2000).

> **CASE STUDY** *continued*
>
> More remote patients are less likely to have their stomach, breast and colorectal cancer diagnosed, and have poorer survival after diagnosis for prostate and lung cancer (Campbell et al., 2000). Another study (Campbell et al., 2001) lends support to the theory that remote/rural patients may be disadvantaged in the early diagnosis of cancer.
>
> * How may interprofessional working address this as an issue?
> * How may nurses develop their roles to better meet the needs of rural patients?

The British Medical Association (BMA, 2005) was concerned enough about this as an issue to resolve in its 2003 meeting to investigate further rural issues and their impact on medical practice. It was particularly interested in the difficulties in recruiting and retaining doctors in rural practices. Concern was expressed particularly about the sustainability of services in rural areas and the resulting problems with access to healthcare.

In a previous report on the nature of rural general practice in the UK, written by the General Practitioners Committee (GPC) of the BMA and the Institute of Rural Health (IRH), four key issues in rural general practice were highlighted. Two of these were:

* 'access for patients in rural areas': if the patient can't get to the doctor . . . will a nurse do instead?
* 'issues of dispensing': to which we may add issues around prescribing and the use of non-medical prescribers. This means health professionals other than doctors taking on the traditional medical role of prescribing medications.

We can thus add to the reduction in hospital junior doctor hours concerns about rural healthcare practice that may well spill over into how nurses will be asked to perform in the future.

Sustainability, climate change and health

Climate change (is) the public health challenge of the 21st century and will come to dwarf all others.

(Griffiths, 2007)

The issues so far discussed have shaped the healthcare context and policy developments. However, health policy (and therefore the work of nurses) in all likelihood will have to face a much sterner challenge. There is a crisis for the continued health of individuals and populations, and this crisis is very probably caused by anthropogenic climate change (Hanson et al., 2007; IPCC, 2007) and unsustainable patterns of living (Schumacher, 1973, 1993; Orr, 1994; Sinclair, 2009). This crisis is deep-seated and has the potential to affect the health and well-being of everyone on the planet (McMicheal and Powells, 1999; DH, 2008a, 2008b; BMA, 2008; Costello et al., 2009) in such a way as to call into question the survival, if not of the human species as a whole, of great swathes of civilisations as we currently understand them. To adapt to and mitigate the effects of climate change, there will be a need to address 'sustainability' (Sustainable Development

Commission (SDC), 2009) in an attempt to reduce Co2 emissions and to ensure that we secure a healthy future for coming generations. Nursing has long considered itself to be about promoting health, not just of individuals but also by implication of wider society. This is implied by nursing's professional body, the NMC, which states:

> *In keeping with the orientation towards holistic care, the emphasis must be one that avoids a narrow disease-orientated perspective and instead encompasses a health promotion and health education perspective.*

(NMC 2004, p14)

Of the many global challenges to health, climate change and unsustainable lifestyles are arguably the most important factors in determining the future health of populations. It may be argued that there needs to be a shift in ideas within nursing, from individualistic, narrowly defined training and biomedical models, towards a more radical ecocentric paradigm (Kleffel, 2004; Goodman and Richardson, 2010). In addition, sustainability is now a policy objective of the UK government (DH, 2008c). This is supported by the Climate Change Act 2008, which makes it the duty of the Secretary of State to ensure that the net UK carbon emissions for all CO_2 equivalent gases for the year 2050 is at least 80 per cent lower than the 1990 baseline. There is, therefore, a legal requirement to address carbon emissions in the UK.

Sustainable living entails ensuring that current patterns of consumption do not endanger the physical resource base (i.e. the planet) or the 'emotional' resource base for coming generations. Human health is based on some fundamentals of the physical environment (clean air, clean water, sufficient food and safe waste disposal) and also upon some fundamentals of the psycho-social environment. A sense of the aesthetic and notions of what constitutes the 'good life' for human happiness cannot be ignored when assessing human health. The latter may not be as clear-cut as the physical needs for health. However, the difficulty in defining what the aesthetic is should not deter us from including it in discussions around sustainable living. Nursing in its holistic sense has to address this if it wishes to clarify what health may mean. Nursing models do highlight this holistic approach, but often focus on the individual rather than as analyses at the philosophical social, political and environmental level. It has been suggested that the responsibility of healthcare practitioners to protect and promote the health of the public should be extended to working to prevent climate change (Gill et al., 2007).

One initiative aimed at enabling people and organisations in the NHS and wider community to engage in activities that support sustainability is 'The Convergence of Health and Sustainable Development'. This is a network of health and other professionals committed to promoting sustainable development within the NHS. This group has proposed a manifesto with a commitment to promoting sustainable development in the NHS and the wider community, and to strengthening the position of sustainable development within the NHS workforce. Signatories to the manifesto include the Faculty of Public Health of the Royal Colleges of Physicians of the UK, the Scottish Environmental Protection Agency, and the UK Public Health Association, as well as a number of senior public health academics and NHS managers. To support this, the Climate Connection website (see below) has been created to bring together interested parties.

The sustainability and climate change agenda means that nurses of the future will have to broaden their understanding of who it is they are working for and with. This may include the idea of global citizenship (Lagos, 2009) and the health of not just humans but of the planet itself.

The climate connection

There is a need for urgent action on climate change for the following reasons.

- Mitigation (reducing greenhouse gas emissions) is not only essential for the long-term protection of public health, but offers huge synergies with health improvement – through promoting physical activity, healthy diet, community development, efficient housing and better air quality.
- Projected climate variability should be properly risk-managed by health and social care services, and in emergency planning. Measures to increase resilience to climate change also offer opportunities for health improvement and reducing inequalities.
- There is now a public health partnership link for members of the nursing, midwifery and healthcare professions, open to all to assist with these aims. This partnership runs the Climate Connection website and forum.

Conclusion

Current health policies have not developed without influence from previous thinking. An historical perspective illustrates how ideas about collaboration have supported current initiatives. It is clear that, in the drive for cost-effective care, better and more integrated services, patient-focused services and the promotion of collaborative practices between professionals, new demands are being placed on all who work in a constantly changing NHS. Nurses have been seen as a key professional group in delivering the new NHS. Much political rhetoric has been published about these various processes. What is now required is more research to see how and if the competing demands and changes are positively affecting the quality of the patient experience. Your task will be to understand that changes are going on around you and to recognise the role of the nurse in collaborating and coordinating relationships with a wide range of professional and non-professional groups.

The main message is that of involving the public in all aspects of health service design and delivery. How you help this process will vary according to your role and clinical setting.

C　　H　　A　　P　　T　　E　　R　　　　　S　　U　　M　　M　　A　　R　　Y

This chapter introduced the background to current policy. You need to understand what the professional body of nursing says about what it means to 'work with others', what influences (historical and political) have shaped thinking and how health policies drive thinking and practice in the National Health Service (NHS). You need to grasp that your work is influenced a great deal by people who are not nurses, and that issues that arise in wider society affect how nurses are asked to go about their daily business. You will note that collaboration, and the lack of it, and the need to listen to the patient's voice have become important issues for the health service to deal with. You will also note that the Department of Health has been very active, especially since 1997, issuing policy documents to reform the NHS. It is partly this political background that has shaped the modern context within which nurses work.

Activities: brief outline answers

Activity 2.1: Evidence-based practice and research (page 28)

- Care, dignity, protect, health, well being, high standards, honesty, integrity, profession.
- Using the preferred name of the patient instead of 'love' or 'dearie'.
- Acting with personal honesty according to one's personal and professional, ethical beliefs. So, agreeing with a professional principle that there ought to be respect between colleagues but then engaging in gossip.
- Nursing has a reputation for putting the needs of patients first, that nurses are as motivated by the need to care for the health of patients before their own personal gain. It has been argued that taking industrial action would challenge the notion of 'public service first'.

Activity 2.2: Critical thinking and group work (page 30)

- A service provider may be a Doctor's Surgery.
- A commissioner may be a Primary Care Trust.
- The design of a service may include the range of services available such as a 'Well Man clinic', and what that service actually looks like in its provision. For example, a Well Man clinic could be doctor or nurse led and may offer cholesterol checking.
- Delivery is, of course, the way that service is provided and may include, for example, the opening hours of a Well Man clinic (this may be five days a week or only every other Saturday).
- Evaluation – how well is the service working, how do you know how well it is working, do you ask patients for their views, have you measurable targets to meet?

To identify how the public and staff are engaged in design, delivery and evaluation, you will need to go into practice and find out!

Activity 2.4: Evidence-based practice and research (page 36)

- See 'Minister accuses doctors over super-surgery petition'. The Guardian, 12 June 2008. www.guardian.co.uk/uk/2008/jun/12/health.nhs
- PFI: The private finance initiative (PFI) provides a way of funding major capital investments, without immediate recourse to the public purse. Private consortia, usually involving large construction firms, are contracted to design, build, and in some cases manage new projects. Contracts typically last for 30 years, during which time the building is leased by a public authority. This section of the site gives guidance to contractors and DH staff on contracts, current news and updates, as well as facts, figures and further information. www.dh.gov.uk Visit the Department of Health website for a full discussion. For an opposing view, see the Unison website: http://www.unison.org.uk/pfi/nhs_intro.asp

Activity 2.5: Evidence-based practice and research (page 37)

1. WHO is the directing and coordinating authority for health within the United Nations system. It is responsible for providing leadership on global health matters, shaping the health research agenda, setting norms and standards,

articulating evidence-based policy options, providing technical support to countries, and monitoring and assessing health needs.
2. The WHO is based in Geneva.
3. The World Health Assembly is the supreme decision-making body for WHO. It meets each year in May and is attended by delegations from all 193 member states. The Executive Board is composed of 34 members technically qualified in the field of health. Members are elected for three-year terms. The main Board meeting, at which the agenda for the forthcoming Health Assembly is agreed upon and resolutions are adopted for forwarding to the Health Assembly, is held in January, with a second shorter meeting in May, immediately after the Health Assembly, for more administrative matters.
4. It is funded by the United Nations and its member states.
5. For the ten key points, see: http://www.who.int/hpr/NPH/docs/declaration_almaata.pdf

Activity 2.6: Critical thinking (page 39)

- This relates to the allocation of very specific roles and tasks to the different occupational groups. For example, it was the case that taking a blood pressure from a patient was the doctor's role and no other professional group was deemed capable of undertaking it. It is necessary to write this because there may be a tendency for professionals to think that particular activities can only be done by specialist groups. This is due to the education and training required to carry out that task. In a patient-led service it may be the case that it should be patient need not availability of staff that steers what can and cannot be done. The prescribing of medicines has always been the preserve of the doctor on this basis. Is it the case that taking a blood sample will be carried out now by a range of occupational groups? Are counselling skills being learned more widely?

Activity 2.9: Critical thinking (page 46)

- Different methods used to access users' views include surveys, focus groups,membership of health committees and public meetings. Can you think of any others?
- To fully explore answers to questions 2, 3 and 4 you need to take them into clinical settings and ask for actual examples of how user involvement is encouraged and delivered. You may wish to discuss this with mentors or tutors.

Activity 2.10: Critical thinking (page 48)

1. The study cannot be generalised as it involves interviewing 59 users who are possibly not representative of the whole population of users. However, if we understand the background in which the study took place we learn a principle that could in theory be applied or checked in another setting.
2. For example, NHS culture may need to change from assuming the professionals know best to one where the service users voice is valued. This would be 'meaningful' as it may actually affect the patient experience.
3. A common theme to be explored in both studies is 'Paternalistic attitudes held by professional groups'. See chapter4.

Knowledge review

Now that you've worked through the chapter, how would you rate your knowledge of the following topics?

	Good	Adequate	Poor
1. The historical context of policy.			
2. Drivers for working together.			
3. Choice and consumerism			

Where you are not confident in your knowledge of a topic, what will you do next?

Further reading

Barrett, G, Sellman, D and Thomas, J (2005) *Interprofessional Working in Health and Social Care.* Basingstoke: Palgrave Macmillan, especially Chapter 1.
This text builds on themes developed in the text and prepares for further chapters.

Day, J (2006) *Interprofessional Working.* Cheltenham: Nelson Thornes, especially Chapter 2.
This text outlines the core ideas around interprofessional working.

Elliott, L and Atkinson D (2007) *Fantasy Island: Waking up to the incredible economic, political and social illusions of the Blair legacy.* London: Constable, especially Chapter 6: The tottering empire state and the crisis in the public sector.
This text is an indulgence read for those of you with an interest in the wider politics of the UK.

Williamson, G, Jenkinson, T and Proctor-Childs, T (2010) *The Contexts of Contemporary Nursing.* Exeter: Learning Matters, especially Chapter 1.
This chapter, on the origins of the NHS, is a must read.

Useful websites

http://theclimateconnection.org A public health base for information and action on sustainability and health.

www.dh.gov.uk For all policy documents on the NHS. Follow links or search within the site for specific topics such as LiNks, PALS, PFI.

www.nhs.uk The NHS home site.

www.nhs.uk/tools/pages/nhstimeline.aspx A history of the NHS from 1948 to the present day. An interactive timeline with milestones.

Chapter 3

The elements of working together: structure, process and culture

Draft NMC Standards for Pre-registration Nursing Education

This chapter will address the following draft competencies:

Domain: Communication and interpersonal skills

1. All nurses must communicate safely and effectively to forge partnerships and build therapeutic relationships with people, family members and groups. They must take individual differences, capabilities and needs into account, and respond in a non-discriminatory way.

Domain: Leadership, management and team working

2. All nurses must work as independent practitioners as well as part of a team, taking a leadership role in co-ordinating, delegating and supervising care safely and appropriately while remaining accountable.

7. All nurses must use their own initiative and practise autonomously and assertively, either as an individual practitioner or as part of a team, managing and prioritising competing demands and, where appropriate, acting as an agent of change to enhance and improve quality of care. They must be able to negotiate effectively and influence others to provide the best care.

Draft Essential Skills Clusters

This chapter will address the following draft ESCs:

Cluster: Organisational aspects of care

14. People can trust the newly registered graduate nurse to be autonomous and confident as a member of the multi-disciplinary or multi-agency team and to inspire confidence in others.

By second progression point:

ii. Supports and assists others appropriately.
iii. Values others' roles and responsibilities within the team and interacts appropriately.
iv. Reflects on own practice and discusses issues with other members of the team to enhance learning.

> **Draft Essential Skills Clusters continued**
>
> *By entry to the register:*
> vi.   Actively consults and explores solutions and ideas with others to enhance care.
> vii. Challenges the practice of self and others across the multi-professional team.
> viii. Takes effective role within the team adopting the leadership role when appropriate.
> x.   Works inter-professionally and autonomously as a means of achieving optimum outcomes for people.

> **Chapter aims**
>
> **After reading this chapter you will be able to:**
>
> * identify the three elements needed for collaborative working;
> * understand the role and importance of culture;
> * recognise how norms, values, beliefs and attitudes affect behaviour;
> * understand socialisation and professional identity.

Introduction

The success of 'working with other people' can be seen to rest (among other things) on the following concepts (Hornby and Atkins, 2000).

* **Structure** – defined as physical, concrete 'things' such as buildings, computer hardware and other equipment. This also includes the personnel and their training, knowledge and skills.
* **Process** – how healthcare is provided. It is more an abstract depiction of the relationship people have with one another: an interconnected flow of information between professionals, or the experiences and the communication they have with a patient as the patient experiences their illness and recovery. It may also be the types of services provided (Family Planning services at a GP surgery, for example), or various treatment options (see 'Early intervention for psychosis' in the box below).
* **Culture** – the values, norms and attitudes held by individuals that may be shaped by the working role they hold.

This chapter will examine each of these in more detail and ask you to reflect on your role in developing and maintaining these elements. You are also required to understand and identify the role of others by working with other professionals. It is suggested that without an understanding of professional cultures there will be opportunities for misunderstanding. Teamworking is based on a clear understanding of our roles and how we learn to be professionals will impact on our ability to be team players. You will also understand that there are elements other than the personal which will also affect this process.

Structure and process

A middle-aged man starts to feel a severe pain in his chest. There is a need to visit a healthcare facility, or call for an ambulance for pain relief, assessment and treatment.

The *structure* of an A & E department should provide, among other things, equipment to give a diagnosis and treatment for a heart attack. The structure of a minor injury unit may not have the same level of sophisticated equipment. The physical structure of the A & E department houses A & E consultants, registrars, staff-grade doctors, nurses, radiographers, etc. The structure of the minor injury unit may house a doctor (but many times does not) and one or two nurses and support workers. The structure of an emergency ambulance is the vehicle itself and all its equipment. The personnel would be the ambulance technician or paramedic. Therefore, how a healthcare setting is structured will make it easier or more difficult for professionals to collaborate. In Chapter 2 we noted how 'telemedicine structures', for example, could bring about more effective and efficient care by improving communication between professionals.

The *process* for dealing with this patient will be different in these three places. There might be a nurse-led process in two cases – the patient may be seen and treated by a nurse practitioner, or seen by a doctor, or indeed both. Who sees the patient first may be the result of clear management direction of the process, or luck, but may well be different in both places. In the case of ambulance paramedics, the process is quite clear – they are the first to see and assess the patient. The professionals will also refer to processes such as the Advanced Cardiac Life Support (ACLS) algorithms as published by the United Kingdom Resuscitation Council in the event of a cardiac arrest. The ACLS process also assumes cooperation between healthcare professionals.

Mental health 'processes': early intervention for psychosis

Marshall and Rathbone (2004) undertook an analysis examining the various treatment options for schizophrenia. For our purposes, what this illustrates is that there exists various 'processes' (treatment options) for what is a relatively common condition.

> *Schizophrenia typically begins in young adulthood and may lead to disability that lasts a lifetime. The onset of psychosis is usually preceded by a period of non-psychotic symptoms, known as prodromal symptoms. The symptoms of full-blown schizophrenia include hallucinations, delusions, disordered thinking, and emotional withdrawal. There is some evidence that a delay in receiving adequate treatment reduces the chances or the extent of recovery.*
>
> (www.cochrane.org/reviews)

Supporters of *early intervention* have argued that outcomes might be improved if more therapeutic efforts were focused on the early stages of schizophrenia or on people with prodromal symptoms. Early intervention in schizophrenia has two elements that are distinct from standard care:

- 'early detection';
- 'phase-specific treatment', which includes medications, cognitive behavioural therapy (CBT) and/or family therapy and/or outpatient care trials. A Scandinavian trial involved 'assertive community treatment' plus family therapy, social skills training and a modified medication regime.

The result of the analysis identified insufficient trials to draw any definitive conclusions about what works best. The substantial international interest in early intervention offers an opportunity to make major positive changes in psychiatric practice, but making the most of this opportunity requires a concerted international programme of research to address key unanswered questions.

Note here that there are a number of intervention options – *processes* – that a client may experience, many of which would mean the professionals' need to collaborate to get the best effective treatment regime. The psychiatrist who prescribes medications must collaborate with the Cognitive Behavioural Therapist to evaluate the success of the prescription medications.

Effects of structure and process

How do structure and process affect people? It is possible to build, design and finance structures that either bring professionals together in one 'space' or to keep them separate. Thus, if the goal is collaboration, then clearly structures have to be built to help this happen. An example would be to have a health clinic staffed by a range of professional groups (GPs, district nurses, midwives, community psychiatric nurses, physiotherapists) in close proximity, where they can easily access patient information and enter into 'real time' discussion about care needs. Ideally, this should reduce the need always to refer and hence wait for another appointment for the patient. This would mean designing the timing of how patients were seen in clinics to allow time and space for this to happen. If a pregnant woman visited a health clinic for a pre-natal check by a midwife, then this service is enhanced if the midwife has easy access to medical information and/or advice from a doctor on site (or remotely, if telemedicine facilities are in place). This entails designing a service that has the patients' needs in mind before the needs of professionals. Current structures have made it difficult in some cases for patients even to access GP services when it is convenient to the patient. Patient complaints have been increasingly received following the introduction in 2004 of new GP contracts that allowed GPs to opt out of night and weekend working: as Stephanie Bown (2007), of the Medical Protection Society stated: *the out of hours experience is increasingly a source of dissatisfaction for patients* (BBC, 2003). The structure and process, therefore, of patient services in this case not only affects collaboration but is an important indicator of a quality service.

Another example of structure and process change is the introduction of the Single Assessment Process (SAP), which was introduced as part of the NSF for Older People (DH, 2001). The SAP was introduced as part of Standard Two: Person-centred care, and describes *a single assessment process across health and social care* (DH, 2001, p30). The policy is:

> an attempt to elevate standards of assessment, to facilitate information sharing between health and social care in order to improve efficiency and lead to more effective care and to provide greater equality in access to multi-agency services.

> (Dickenson, 2006, p365)

Assessment is a crucial gateway to services across a range of agencies and therefore the skill of the assessor and the assessment process is vital for efficient and effective service delivery to older people in need of health and social care. Professional groups had been used to assessing patients using their own separate documentation, which was not always easily accessible to other professional groups. This also involved duplication of gathering information and presenting it in a way that makes sense for the profession but not always for others.

For example, a medical practitioner may be primarily interested in physiological (biological) information and needs to quickly access information such as blood test results (say, for thyroid function). A physiotherapist, however, may be focused on the patient's mobility needs and does not want to have to wade through pages of medication prescriptions and laboratory results. The challenge for any single documentation and assessment process is to allow both professionals to record and access their information in such a way as to meet the patient's and their own needs.

Activity 3.1   *Evidence-based practice and research*

Mary Brown is an 87-year-old lady and was recently widowed, having been the main carer for her husband. Mary lives in a large Victorian property with coal-fired heating on the outskirts of small town in the North of England. Mary is known to her GP, Dr Young, through caring for her late husband. Her own health has gradually deteriorated since a fall some six months ago while getting her husband out of bed. Mary's daughter, who lives in Manchester, has asked Dr Young to review Mary due to her failing health. Mary is no longer as mentally alert as she was and appears weak and lethargic.

Source: www.cpa.org.uk.

- How will Mary's needs be assessed?
- What services do you think Mary will require?
- What professional (and voluntary) groups may need to be involved?
- How will they know when and what is required?
- Who will make the referrals and what information will that person gather?
- Who will be responsible for the coordination, and evaluation of the success of those services?

For answers to address this activity fully, you may wish to discuss this with a mentor in a community primary care placement.

Dickenson (2006) argues:

Possibly the greatest potential threat to the successful implementation of SAP will be the need for professionals from health and social care to work together.

The boundaries between health and social care have been in existence at least since the modern welfare state was established In England, the boundaries are evidenced by the division of health and social care delivery between separate organisations. Within the National Health Service in England, primary care health services are currently commissioned and managed within Primary Care Trusts (PCTs), while social care services are managed and provided through local councils. Current government policy places a great emphasis on partnership working. Collaborations across health and social care boundaries have been defined as 'a way of working with others on a joint project where there is a shared interest in positive outcomes'. However, inter-agency and interprofessional collaboration have proved to be difficult to achieve in practice. Reasons given for the difficulties include: differing professional perspectives, cultures and poor understanding of professional roles.

(p366)

The structure of a SAP (and the process it requires staff to work through) may not be sufficient on its own to encourage collaboration, but it may be a necessary first step. Dickenson implies that the issue of working together may actually be a problem for professionals and indicates some reason why this is so. The conclusion from this study is:

In order to close the implementation gap for SAP, that is, to reduce the distance between policy objectives and achievements, practitioners working in increasingly pressurised NHS and community care settings need effective support in order to change the way they practise. Practitioners cannot be expected to make this transition unaided and without this support, and are likely to respond by limited or non-participation in the process as seen in this (study) and previous work. The pivotal role given to assessment meant success or otherwise of the reforms lay in part on the ability of practitioners to make this transition.

(p379)

In other words, introducing a structure will not work on its own. Professional culture and practice has to change to make it work.

What goes for structures goes for processes too. If we think of a treatment option as a process, we may understand that there are options and complications. Some processes may mean a lone practitioner; others may demand more closer working between professionals. The mental health example (early intervention for psychosis) demonstrates the complicated treatment options that need to be coordinated. For example, without understanding the goals and methods of CBT, how would a psychiatrist make the best prescription options? One factor that would be taken into account is the way that the drugs prescribed will alter mental states and ways of thinking which may help or hinder the CBT work.

This example may be an ideal type of interprofessional collaboration. If all the elements (structure, process and culture) are 'positively aligned' (that is to say, each supports and reinforces the other), then we may see an improved outcome for the patient (rapid assessment, diagnosis and treatment). If, however, they are negatively aligned, the outcome may be worse.

Unless the nurse is in a senior management position, the opportunity to change the major structure(s) of an organisation will be limited. There may be opportunities, however, to change small structures within clinical areas. When it comes to process, again this may depend on what role the nurse has in the clinical team.

Activity 3.2   *Evidence-based practice and research, and critical thinking*

Discuss with your mentor in practice the meaning of the two terms, 'structure' and 'process'. Illustrate with concrete examples. Try to work out how a patient experiences the processes they have to go through in their illness, recovery or health journey.

Activity 3.2 continued

For example, adolescents – 'teenagers, 11–16 years old' – what *structures* and *processes* exist for dealing with their:

- sex and relationship education (SRE) needs (includes emergency contraception);
- in-hospital surgical/medical treatments;
- suicide risk or depression needs;
- substance abuse issues?

An outline answer is given at the end of the chapter.

Culture

The third aspect of this approach to working with others is the need to understand culture and the dynamics of personal and interpersonal communication. What skills, knowledge and insights will you need to participate successfully in the team? Participation is not only at the level of performing tasks but in helping teams to grow, work more smoothly and to focus on the agreed goals of healthcare, which should include better patient care.

Activity 3.3   *Reflection*

Barrett et al. (2005) have identified the processes required for effective interprofessional working. Their use of the word 'process' may be confusing. It may assist us to think of these things as part of an 'occupational culture' – that is to say, the personal values, norms, attitudes and behaviours that individuals exhibit towards one another such as:

- knowledge of professional roles – knowing what we all do;
- willing participation – a positive attitude that actively seeks cooperation;
- confidence;
- open and honest communication – being clear what you mean;
- having trust and mutual respect between professional groups;
- dealing with power, i.e. dealing with those who can make the influential decisions and who may have their own goals;
- conflict management;
- securing senior management-level support;
- dealing with uncertainty;
- dealing with envy;
- anxiety management.

Reflect on how these skills are acknowledged and developed.

In addition, they suggest several strategies to support interprofessional working:

- engaging in reflection and clinical supervision;
- evaluation of current roles and practices;
- education and training for interprofessional working;

Activity 3.3 continued

- reinforcement of professional identity;
- ensuring managerial support;
- developing realistic expectations.

As the answer will depend on your own observation and experience, there is no outline answer at the end of the chapter.

As was noted in Chapter 2, Elston and Holloway (2001) had interviewed GPs, nurses and practice managers in three Primary Care centres to compare their perspectives on changes to primary care, including moves towards interprofessional collaboration and the development of their professional roles. They identified that *professional identities* and *traditional power structures* generated conflict. They concluded: *it will take a new generation of health professionals to bring about an interprofessional culture in the NHS.* This suggests that 'culture' may negatively affect the working together of healthcare professionals. We will examine professional identity and traditional power structures in Chapter 4. First, we need to understand what we mean by:

- culture;
- occupational culture;
- interprofessional culture.

What is culture?

Culture is:

- the **shared beliefs** and **values** of a group: the beliefs, customs, practices and social behaviour of a particular nation or people;
- **shared attitudes**: a particular set of attitudes that characterises a group of people.
  (http://encarta.msn.com)

You will have come across the notion of culture before. This is not about the arts ('high' culture) but about the shared norms, beliefs, values and attitudes of groups of people. You may well have heard of 'working-class culture' or 'ethnic minority culture'. These terms refer to the widest sense of culture, which involves issues such as language used, the way people dress, the food they eat, what they like as leisure, whether they value work as a means to an end or an end in itself. The description is almost limitless.

Culture thus involves the following shared attributes.

Activity 3.4   *Reflection*

Think about your social group, the people you live and mix with socially. Identify those shared aspects of living that bind you together. Think about what it would be like to be an outsider. What would it be about your lifestyle and attitudes, for example, that they would find difficult to understand?

A brief outline answer is given at the end of the chapter.

Norms

Each social group will have a 'code of conduct'. This may be made very explicit, written down and discussed by everybody or it may be something one has grown up with, forming part of everyday experience. This 'code' decides what is acceptable to the group. It helps to define what makes up 'norms of behaviour', which, if a member does not keep to them, may result in 'sanctions' (positive or negative). Sanctions are brought to bear on an individual (or a group) to make them get 'back in line'. To belong to a group is to know what its norms are.

Norms relate to behaviour often in specific situations. One reason you may feel uncomfortable in a new social setting is that you may not have learned what the norms are for that group in that setting. Consider the norms of behaviour in a typical middle-class English wedding reception.

One way to bring norms to light (those that are so everyday they are taken for granted) is to break them. Howard Garfinkel was a sociologist interested in the everyday experience of social rules and is often accepted as the 'father' of a branch of sociology called 'ethnomethodology' (Garfinkel, 1967; Goodman and Strange, 1997). Garfinkel suggested the disruption (temporarily) of the world that we take for granted to expose the background assumptions (norms, values and beliefs) that have been accepted as reality for a long time. He wished to note people's reaction to this disruption. In one of his experiments Garfinkel asked his students to behave as if they were visitors or 'paying customers' in their own homes. The bemused reactions of their parents were then recorded by the students. The struggle by parents to comprehend the sudden disruption of their informal relationship built up over many years with their children became apparent. The students had stepped out of 'son or daughter' role and assumed the behaviours and role of 'guest'.

Imagine coming down to breakfast in the morning in your own home, all the while taking on the role of 'guest' as if in a hotel. You will have adopted a new set of social norms, which will become very clear if your partner or parents are not privy to your game. This illustrates that unless the individuals or social groups (guest/waiter or spouse-spouse) share the norms, misunderstanding and conflict may arise.

Activity 3.5   **Reflection**

What norms of behaviour apply to members of occupational groups? For example, is it a norm to refer to a medical consultant as 'mate'? Is it a norm for nurses to wear nose studs and, if so, in what context? Are all norms appropriate? Do we need to ask why we behave in certain ways? What ways of speaking to elderly patients or children are deemed acceptable and why?

Many staff may be seen wearing stethoscopes around their necks when in clinical practice settings. This is a 'norm' of behaviour that would look out of place at the breakfast table. Why do staff wear stethoscopes around their necks? Is it only because it is a practical way to carry them? Do norms therefore have certain messages associated with them? Is the wearing of a stethoscope a way of indicating a person's status when they are not wearing a uniform, white coats or operating theatre clothing?

As the answers will be based on your own observations, there is no outline answer at the end of the chapter.

Values

This involves the judgement of something's worth or importance. The 'something' may be an object, activity or an abstract concept such as 'sanctity of life'. Values may be ethical/moral, ideological/political, social, or aesthetic/artistic. Values are judged subjectively by individuals and groups, and one way to uncover them is to note what gets respected or honoured within a group. Thus the values of a society can often be identified by noting which people receive honour or respect. In the United States, for example, are professional athletes more highly honoured than college professors? Is this because US society values physical activity and competitiveness more than mental activity and education? Is financial reward linked to what is valued?

If financial reward *is* linked to what is valued, respected, looked up to, and related to ideas of rarity and preciousness, what do we value in the United Kingdom? What gets financially rewarded? You may wish to argue that we honour and respect using other means of expressing it.

Activity 3.6   *Critical thinking*

Describe the outward mark of respect and honour that society shows towards the differing professions and occupational groups listed below.

- Politicians
- Barristers
- Journalists
- Teachers
- Social workers
- Registered nurses
- Registered midwives
- Engineers
- NHS managers
- 'Blue collar' workers: cleaners, shop workers, van drivers.

If there is a difference in the value given to these occupations, why may that be so?

A brief outline answer is given at the end of the chapter.

You may argue that, in the UK, we also value freedom of expression to wear what we like and freedom of speech to say what we like; we value rights for women to take part in work and political life. Some radical (Wahaabi) Islamist groups value the opposite (Hussein, 2007).

Is success in business, a high salary, a professional career, the ability to control, organise, and create and predict complex processes and organisations; is a long educational experience and its attendant qualifications and entry to a closely controlled professional group valued more than the application of skills and knowledge to domestic activities in the home? Is cure valued more than care? Is prediction valued more than intuition? How is a training for a vocation valued against a professional qualification?

What values are explicitly taught to nurses? What values are rewarded in nursing practice and what values attract negative sanctions? There will be a difference in what we all value, and in clinical practice there may be a difference in what occupational groups value. It is these differences and similarities that will impact on how we work together.

Fahrenwald et al. (2005) argue:

> *Nursing is a caring profession. Caring encompasses empathy for and connection with people. Teaching and role-modelling caring is a nursing curriculum challenge. Caring is best demonstrated by a nurse's ability to embody the five core values of professional nursing. Core nursing values essential to baccalaureate education include human dignity, integrity, autonomy, altruism, and social justice. The caring professional nurse integrates these values in clinical practice.*

This is from the United States' perspective. Identify what the core nursing values may be for the UK.

A brief outline answer is given at the end of the chapter.

Values and health-seeking behaviour

A patient's values may very well affect where they go for therapy and treatment and, in some cases, this will be at odds with a professional group's idea of what works.

Messerli-Rohrbach (2000) undertook a research study into whether patients' spiritual values affected their use of non-conventional medicine. The study aimed to establish whether 'materialistic' or 'post-materialistic' values and spiritual preferences correlated with the use of 'unconventional' (complementary and alternative) medical methods. In other words, are people who have rejected the idea of the acquisition of material possessions as a good thing in itself (post-materialists), more likely to be wary of conventional Western medicine? Do their 'spiritual values' relate to their health-seeking behaviours?

In 1995 and 1996, 3,077 and 2,276 Swiss residents were interviewed by telephone. They were asked about their use of the conventional medical system and also about their views on spirituality and materialism. Results suggested and confirmed that the idea that certain values, attitudes and convictions influence the use of complementary medicine. Post-materialists and interviewees who tended to agree with neoreligious (New Age) statements used complementary medicine significantly more frequently than materialists. Interviewees who tended to disagree with 'neoreligiosity' or who tended towards traditional Christian values were less likely to use complementary medicine.

For our purposes we may think of post-materialists as 'New Age' thinkers – i.e. those who believe in such practices as crystal healing, biofeedback, guided imagery and reiki. For a fuller description of New Age thinking, see Tucker (2004) or Kumar on www.virtuescience.com/newage.html; for healing practices, see the Complementary Healthcare Information Service UK on www.chisuk.org.uk/index.php.

In what way would the approach to understanding and treating depression differ between those who value conventional scientific approaches and those who believe in the effects and value the use of therapies such as reiki and homeopathy?

Activity 3.8 continued

- Are there any values common to New Age healing philosophy and nursing?
- Are there any values common to New Age philosophy and medicine?
- Are there any values common to nursing and medicine?

A brief outline answer is given at the end of the chapter.

Beliefs

Our beliefs are the psychological state in which we are convinced of the truth of a proposition (X is X and not Y, X causes Y, if I do X then Y happens, or X cures Y). They may be based on experience, evidence, prejudice, ancient texts or given to us by parents, schools, peers or worked out by ourselves through study and/or emotion. The evidence upon which we base a belief about the truth of something may come from research, sensory experience, case studies, and practical experience. Closely related to our beliefs are our *opinions* (our ideas and thoughts about something; our assessment, judgement or evaluation of something).

A belief will thus guide opinions, form attitudes and guide action. If you believe that there is a God who punishes sin, and if you believe illness is a punishment from God for your sinning, you may act to avoid this punishment. You may pray to the Almighty to forgive your sins; you may undertake good works to avoid becoming ill. If you become ill you may seek the cause of it in your displeasing of God. Your opinion of someone who does not follow the faith may be low; you may assess them as being misguided, to be pitied and evaluate their lifestyle choices in negative terms.

If you believe 'like cures like', that 'water has memory', that there is a 'single remedy', 'No matter how many symptoms are experienced, only one remedy is taken, and that remedy will be aimed at all those symptoms', you may encourage your friends to do the same because 'it worked for me, the illness was only cured when I started taking the *Arsenicum album*, the *Nux vomica* or the *China officinalis*'. You may thus approach 'traditional' medicine with a critical attitude.

Attitudes

Attitudes may be defined as a disposition or tendency to respond positively or negatively towards ideas, objects, people and/or situations. Attitudes may encompass, or be closely related to, our opinions and beliefs, and are often based on our experiences.

Working with other people involves dealing with the attitudes of others and sometimes attempting to change those attitudes. Hovland et al. (1953) provided one of the first major theories of attitude change, involving 'persuasive communication'. According to Hovland et al.'s theory, *rewards* are linked to attitude change. It is suggested that the learning of new attitudes is no different from any other verbal or motor skill; the acceptance of a new opinion (and hence attitude formation) is dependent on the rewards and incentives offered.

Imagine you are the chief executive of a large organisation. You have this position because of the work you have put in over the years. If holding a certain opinion of yourself in this instance involves feelings of superiority (of intellect or of occupational worth), which may result in an attitude of 'aloofness' towards others who appear not as important, what rewards or incentives would seem to support this sort of opinion and attitude? What rewards and incentives would seem to justify this to yourself? Who bestows these rewards and incentives? In what ways do the 'others' either support or challenge your own opinions and attitudes.

Think: Rewards and incentives are not just the size of one's salary.

As this task is for you to tease out, there is no outline answer at the end of the chapter.

According to Festinger's (1957) theory of cognitive dissonance (CD), a conflict between beliefs causes attitude change.

- **Dissonance** From music, meaning tones or two notes, for example, that sound discordant and need resolution. The two notes are not pleasant to listen to. The listener is uncomfortable with the sound. A musician may wish to play a different note to harmonise – to resolve – the dissonance.
- **Cognition** To do with thoughts and thinking. Therefore, cognitive dissonance is the uncomfortable tension that results from having two conflicting thoughts at the same time. To resolve this dissonance, one of the thoughts has to change.

CD suggests that there is a tendency for individuals to seek consistency among their beliefs and opinions. When there is an *inconsistency between two or more attitudes or beliefs* (this is the 'dissonance'), something must change to eliminate the dissonance.

There may also be a dissonance between attitudes and behaviour. Kearsley (2007) states that, *In the case of a discrepancy between attitudes and behaviour, it is most likely that the attitude will change to accommodate the behaviour.* It is not that simple, however, as a number of factors determine how strong the feelings of 'dissonance' are and therefore how much effort is needed to change attitudes. It does suggest that by dealing with the factors, attitudes can change, they are not fixed. In practice, attitudes may well be almost impossible to change given constraints placed on individuals to alter those factors.

The two main factors that affect how strong the dissonance is felt are the number of dissonant beliefs and the importance attached to each belief.

There are three ways to eliminate dissonance:

1. reduce the importance of the dissonant beliefs;
2. add more consonant (supporting or comfortable) beliefs to outweigh the dissonant beliefs;
3. change the dissonant beliefs so that they are no longer inconsistent.

Kearsley (2007) states:

Dissonance occurs most often in situations where an individual must choose between two incompatible beliefs or actions. The greatest dissonance is created when the two alternatives are equally attractive.

For example, consider someone who buys an expensive pair of shoes (to add to an ever-growing collection), but then discovers that they are not comfortable to walk in for more than 10–15 minutes (the heels may be too high). Dissonance exists between their beliefs that they have bought 'really nice shoes' and that nice shoes should at least get them through an evening without the need for calling an ambulance. Dissonance could be eliminated by deciding that it does not matter since the shoes are mainly used for short dinner parties (reducing the importance of the dissonant belief) or focusing on the shoes' expense, looks, envious and admiring glances from peers and dinner guests (thereby adding more beliefs that support the original decision). The dissonance could also be eliminated by getting rid of the shoes, but this behaviour is a lot harder to achieve than changing beliefs.

Cognitive dissonance for a children's nurse

A children's nurse may hold general beliefs about children as being in need of protection, as starting out in life as innocents, incapable of evil, malicious acts of violence, threat, abuse or self-mutilation, but, after visiting a children's secure unit as part of a continuing professional development course into substance abuse, discovers that children can commit arson or an assault and can kill. Her professional life so far has brought her into contact with the 'normal' child who needs medical or surgical intervention. Her own 'nice' upbringing has so far shielded her from the Dickensian social conditions that some children are brought up in. The James Bulger case (a two-year-old toddler abducted and murdered by two ten-year-olds in 1993) was an aberration, and, though terrible, did not affect her emotionally in any lasting way due to time and distance.

Dissonance exists for this nurse because the picture of the 'child' she holds in her head is contradicted by the stories of the children in front of her in the secure unit. Conflict exists between her belief of 'child as innocent' and now her belief of 'the venal (corruptible, corrupted) child'. How can children be both?

Dissonance can be resolved by deciding that this negative view of the child does not matter because it is so rare and is a product of disordered upbringing, and that at least these children are secure and cannot harm anyone else. Thus the importance of the dissonant belief is reduced because it is contained within a particular environment, it does not apply to the children she will care for.

Dissonance could be countered by adding consonant beliefs – beliefs that support more normal ideas of children and downplaying the negatives, possibly through denying the existence of childhood in the children who she sees before her. A line of reasoning could be that these are no longer children because of their particular experiences and actions, and as sad as that is, this accounts for their behaviour. They cannot be children because children 'don't do those things'. The image of the venal child can be wiped from her mind by definition.

The need to demonise, to distance a child from our accepted notions of what a child is, was illustrated in the Bulger case. One of his killers was known as 'the one who did not cry', while *Detectives who interviewed him following his arrest described him as canny, intelligent and frightening. They were unnerved by his failure to react like a confused child, and some came to hate him, regarding him with a contempt usually reserved for sex criminals and adult child killers* (Kelso, 2001). Maybe society felt a collective dissonance between its notions of childhood and the facts of James Bulger's killing, which led to relabelling the child killers as almost adult.

Behaviour

As we have seen in the discussion of norms of behaviour, there are positive and negative sanctions for 'deviation' from the norm. Behaviour is, of course, bound up with your beliefs, values, and your opinions and attitudes. It often refers to the action (or reaction) of a person usually to external environmental stimuli or through internal thought processes. It can thus be conscious, unconscious, overt, covert, voluntary ('I chose to do it') or involuntary ('he made me do it'). It is with the seen, concrete, tangible behaviours that we have to deal with as soon as we are in groups. The hidden aspects are usually off-limits in our everyday existence. The unconscious mind (as far as we know) has no material existence other than the physical brain and is unknown even to the holder of that consciousness. Thus the unconscious elements of behaviour are by definition almost impossible to fathom.

There are various theoretical perspectives of understanding (and changing) human behaviour. They range from the behaviourist school and cognitive theories through to psychodynamic theory (Gross and Kinnison, 2007).

Cognitive Behavioural Therapy is an attempt to change conscious ways of thinking and thus to alter long-established behaviour patterns. However, we may put forward the view that the outward appearance of behaviour may have its roots in attitudes, values and beliefs that may be unknown to the 'actor'.

Psychoanalysis (Freud, Jung) is an attempt to uncover the unconscious basis for behaviour and conscious thoughts. Psychodynamic theories (such as transactional analysis) attempt to explain behaviour in these terms. Psychoanalysis has been criticised as a 'pseudoscience' (Borch Jacobson, 2005) because it cannot be verified or refuted in the real world of material existence. Nonetheless, it remains popular in some healthcare settings as a way of dealing with deep-seated human consciousness.

Occupational culture and socialisation

We have noted previously that successful interprofessional working involves getting the three elements of structure, process and culture working together, and so far we have noted that culture can involve the elements of:

- norms;
- values;
- beliefs and attitudes;
- behaviour.

These elements apply to general culture but may also apply to the culture of an *occupational group*.

We have seen that culture is a complicated concept, and that in its widest sense it involves just about everything we do. In the healthcare setting, does the idea of occupational culture assist us in understanding how we work together? The examples from above have indicated that it does. There is benefit to be had from examining the notion of 'occupational culture' in a little more detail. This also leads us to discuss a related idea, socialisation, for when we understand these ideas we may begin to see why groups act, speak and interact as they do.

The key questions will be:

- Are nurses socialised in such a way as to challenge the ideals of nursing?
- Are professional groups socialised into their professions in such a way as to make interprofessional working more difficult?

- Are patients socialised into a particular way of interacting with healthcare professionals and services? And if so, in what ways?

Socialisation

We may understand the idea that we are born into a society that has certain *rules* of behaviour and we, as human beings, *learn* these rules through a process of socialisation. *Socialisation* simply means the various ways we learn how to be a human being and are taught the basic rules of the society in which we live. In this respect, one of the central ideas of sociology is that people are not born knowing how to behave. If this is true, it means people must, in effect, learn how to 'be human'. When it comes to joining an occupational group we have a new set of rules to learn. Becoming a nurse is not just about learning the science and art of nursing practice. It is often about learning the unvoiced rules.

Occupational socialisation (Watson, 2003) refers to ways in which people 'learn the ropes' (a term derived from the Royal Navy, whereby new sailors had to name and understand how to use the ropes on a sailing ship). Sociologists have been interested in this process for a while. Becker et al. (1976) described medical students' developing common perspectives or 'modes of thought and action' as they learn the transition from learner to physician.

The process is quite complex with some writers (Luke, 2003) criticising the notion of socialisation for suggesting that people are only passive receivers of norms and the social rules. The process should also be seen as one of action, where people actively create the social world in which they live. However, there must be an acknowledgement of the idea of power and constraint. After all, students of nursing and medicine are not completely free to make up the knowledge base and habits of the profession, particularly in their early careers.

Goldenberg and Iwasiw (1993) define this process as:

> A complex interactive process by which the content of the professional role (skills, knowledge, behaviour) is learned, and the values, attitudes and goals integral to the profession and sense of occupational identity which are characteristic of a member of that profession are internalised.
>
> (p4)

The word 'internalised' refers to the way in which this learning becomes 'internal' – i.e. becomes part of who you are – and may not be conscious. Think of internalising driving skills. Many times you will have arrived at your destination without being consciously aware of actually driving the car.

Melia (1984, 1987) further suggested that professions do not have one overarching set of beliefs and values, but rather have 'segments'. In the case of nursing, the two main segments are 'education' (promoting the professionalisation of nursing) and 'service' (getting the work done), each differently defining *what* work should be done and *how* it should be done. The education segment is largely located within higher education institutions (when Melia wrote her piece, education was located within the NHS in schools of nursing). Service is located within NHS settings, hospital Trusts, and Primary Care Trusts, and is primarily focused on delivering healthcare services to patients and clients. Both have a responsibility for producing the next generation of health workers. Higher education has, of course, a research focus as well as a teaching focus, which further creates the possibility of setting up potentially competing versions of pro-fessional nursing to learner nurses.

This creates a problem for students of nursing who are being socialised into the profession. The classic 'theory–practice' gap here is that what is being taught in education may not be the same as what is being done in practice. In addition, educational priorities may well be different from service priorities. Therefore, what occurs is not a clean process of learning the appropriate ways of behaving and acting.

Mackintosh (2006) argues that the consequences of this form of occupational socialisation for nurses have included:

- lack of critical awareness of practice;
- continuance of ritualised practices;
- the importance of an assumed set of professional characteristics;
- the loss of idealism on behalf of the students.

Ford and Walsh (1990) discussed the reasons for failures on the part of the nursing profession to reach the standards expected by society in relation to the application of research. They described the rituals and myths that abounded in hospital wards that hamper progress in nursing care. Occupational socialisation may account for the reason why this continues as Mackintosh highlights ritualised practice in the later research.

Research summary

Mackintosh (2006) investigated the impact of socialisation on student nurses' ability to care. This was a longitudinal qualitative study of a purposive sample of pre-registration student nurses undergoing an Advanced Diploma Programme at a university in the UK.

- 16 student nurses took part, with 13 completing both stages of data collection.
- Data was collected at 6–9 months after commencing training, and then 18 months later, 6–9 months prior to completing the course.
- Data was collected using tape-recorded semi-structured interviews.

The socialisation process (echoing Melia's work) has not always been positive. It tended to lead to an apparent and relative desensitisation of some student nurses to human need. This reflects perhaps the competing ideas and working practices that students are exposed to. This may be a result of cognitive dissonance as students struggle to resolve conflicting ideas of what it is to be a nurse. The study further argues that this is a result of:

- prior unrealistic expectations of nursing;
- exposure to poor role models that devalue personal care;
- sudden exposure to the emotional demands of the role they are unable to cope with.

These findings are at odds with the large body of literature that emphasises the importance of care and caring activities within nursing. This results in an inherent contradiction between nursing as a caring profession and the actual work that nurses are socialised to perform. Mackintosh describes the changes experienced by students in terms of coping, fears, hardness and disillusionment, and concludes that the result has been largely negative:

- loss of humanitarian ideals is a common thread, with some individual variability;
- this is strongly linked to the need to care less in order to cope more with the work of the nurse.

Compare this view with your earlier identification of core nursing values. This illustrates the changing, dynamic nature of learning a profession and the very personal nature of the work. Working with other people, therefore, is the core of many nurses' perceptions of themselves and the profession. This also leads us to think about how other professionals socialise its members, and the set of attitudes, values and beliefs that result.

Thus, students undertake a transition from naive neophyte to a (hardened?) professional. Benner's (1984) description of novice (the need to follow explicit rules) to expert nurse (the use of intuition and deeply learned skills) may describe how nurses think in relation to the application of their skills and knowledge but may miss important elements – i.e. it may be a naive description of how nurses actually work.

Working with other people therefore involves managing transitions within your own profession as much as learning what it means to work with other professional groups and patients.

Professional identity and social identity theory

Adams et al. (2006) argue that social identity theory may be useful to understand the development of professional identity. The theory suggests that a group's behaviour and attitudes towards another is heavily influenced by the strength of the group's own identity and the relevance of that identify to the group. It is further suggested (Adams et al., 2006) that professional identity is one form of social identity as it:

> concerns group interactions in the workplace and relates to how people compare and differentiate themselves from other professional groups. Professional identity develops over time and involves gaining insight into professional practices and the development of the talents and the values of the profession. It can be described as the attitudes, values, knowledge, beliefs and skills that are shared with others within a professional group and relates to the professional role being undertaken by the individual, and thus is a matter of the subjective self-conceptualization associated with the work role adopted.
>
> (p56)

Primarily established by Henri Tajfel (1974) and his colleagues in the early 1970s, this theory asserts that we must do more than study the psychology of individuals as individuals, but must understand how, when and why individuals define themselves in terms of their group memberships and how these memberships as a consequence effect the behaviour of employees within organisations.

Concept summary continued

Tajfel found that even when individuals were grouped in terms of the most trivial of criteria (e.g. their preference for abstract painters), group members displayed in-group favouritism by awarding more points to in-group members.

Individuals were found to display this bias even when by doing so they reduced their own individual economic gain. From these studies Tajfel concluded that this process of categorising oneself as a group member gives an individual's behaviour a distinct meaning, creating a positively valued social identity.

This group identity then becomes an integral aspect of an individual's sense of 'who they are'.

As a consequence of this new-found identity, individuals want to see 'us' as different from and better than 'them' and hence display in-group favouritism in order to enhance self-esteem.

Source: F Bellanca (Exeter University), www.teambuilding.co.uk/social_identity_theory.html.

Cohen (1981) argues:

learning to be a physician becomes a very important part of one's self concept and a bolster to one's self-esteem. Our society permits subordinating all other relevant roles to the professional identity. The higher the status of the profession, the more this process of subordinating all other relevant roles will be allowed.

(p177)

An individual's sense of who they are may very well depend on the context in which they find themselves. A woman at home, preparing breakfast for herself while supervising her children who are getting ready for school, experiences the individual identity of 'mother'. If the children are young enough to require pre-school care and supervision in a crèche the same woman, on taking the children to the crèche and meeting other mothers, may very well experience the shared group identity of 'mother'. The theory suggests that there will be an unvoiced understanding, for example, of the joys and challenges of child rearing. There may well be a subjective feeling of 'bonding' (although this may be temporary) with other mothers of young children.

This same woman may well be undertaking an education course which leads to a professional qualification. When the context changes, from home or crèche, to education or clinical practice, the group identity changes. The subjective feeling may now be orientated to a new group of 'students of nursing/medicine/physiotherapy'. Cohen's argument suggests that, if this woman is a medical student, the new professional identity will be the stronger identity.

Activity 3.10   *Reflection*

- How would you describe the group identity of student nurses and of a registered nurses?
- How is the group identity of student nurses outwardly expressed by group members?
- How do students of nursing learn what the group identity is?
- How strong is your identity as a student nurse?

Activity 3.10 continued

- How relevant is your student nurse identity to your own sense of who you are?
- How do you express your own nursing identity?
- How do the general public express their view of the professional identity of nurses?

As this task is for you to take back into your own experience and to identify examples, there is no outline answer at the end of the chapter,

What this all suggests is that members of professional groups have learned an identity and a set of attitudes, behaviours, values and norms that may be quite different from those identities experienced by others. Therefore, this is a factor that needs to be taken into account when professional groups are asked to work together. Adams et al. (2006) suggest that a degree of professional identity already exists even *before* students begin their studies.

If professional identity means that individuals will define themselves (*be biased towards – with 'in-group' favouritism*) by their profession, does this imply that collaboration will be more difficult? If the professional cultures are different, where are the common points of agreement? Where are the points of misunderstanding and conflict? Read the extract from the study by Anita Atwal and Kay Caldwell. Is this an example of professional cultures clashing? Why are nurses and social workers reluctant to voice their opinion in team meetings? Why did the medical consultant give more opinions? Is there something about the way nurses and social workers learn to be professionals? Is conformity in a group more highly valued in these groups (as part of their identity) than challenging? Is this study further evidence of a hierarchy in professional standing rather than true collaboration?

Research summary

In 'Do all health and social care professionals interact equally? A study of interactions in multidisciplinary teams in the United Kingdom', Atwal and Caldwell (2005) argue:

> Problems around deficits in interprofessional collaboration have been identified since the National Health Service (NHS) was introduced. It is within the context of the current policy focus on improving collaborative working that this study was undertaken. A direct observational study was carried out in two older persons teams to explore patterns of interaction in the multidisciplinary team meetings. Analysis revealed some key differences in the way in which different professions interacted. Occupational therapists, physiotherapists, social workers (SW) and nurses rarely asked for opinions and for orientation. The consultant (the individual in charge of the medical team) tended to have high rates for asking for orientation, giving opinions and giving orientation. Although some nurses did have high individual rates for the giving of orientation. The data from the research has highlighted that therapists, SWs and nurses are reluctant to voice their opinions in multidisciplinary teams and thus conformity may

Research summary continued

> *dominate its culture. It is suggested that therapists, SWs and nurses need to cite their opinions in teams more effectively if they are to be competent and committed patient-centred practitioners.*
>
> (p268)

Conclusion

Working together involves combining the three elements of structure, process and culture. Each element is challenging and nurses will play different roles in each. This will require the development of specific skills, understandings and knowledge. The professional culture of nursing and other professions will greatly affect this process. We may ask how ready nurses are to take on the challenge as outlined in, for example, *Making a Difference* (DH, 1999)? Is there anything in professional nursing culture that helps this process along?

In the next chapter we will examine in depth the key working relationship between the two main professional groups in the NHS – nurses and doctors.

C H A P T E R S U M M A R Y

This chapter introduced the idea that successful collaborative practice rests on the three elements of structure, process and culture, with special emphasis on culture. You will note the obvious point that working with people means understanding *how* people work! It is important to understand that concrete things such as equipment, buildings and funding may constrain what we do and how we do it. It is also important to grasp how 'systems' have been designed to get work done. It is arguably more important to note how people as social beings shape these concrete entities, abstract processes and their social relationships. It is the daily decisions, values, norms, attitudes and beliefs (our 'culture'), for example, that have enormous influence on the experiences of those in working environments.

Activities: brief outline answers

Activity 3.2: Evidence-based practice and research, and critical thinking (pages 66–7)

- Substance abuse treatments. Specific interventions include in-patient programmes, out-patient programmes, 'therapeutic community' type of programmes, and outward bound or life skills training type of programmes. On-site group counselling programmes can be provided by schools. See also 'Talk to Frank' www.talktofrank.com/home_html.aspx
- See 'Every Child Matters' www.everychildmatters.gov.uk/

Activity 3.4: Reflection (page 68)

There are almost as many examples of this as there are groups and individuals. However, a very common experience is that of adolescence and early adulthood. Teenagers are often seeking their own identity and in doing so bond with peers to establish modes of speech and dress that leave older generations perplexed. Take text messaging, any examination of who engages in this and the manner in which they do it demonstrates the membership or otherwise of particular social groupings.

Activity 3.6: Critical thinking (page 70)

Society shows respect and honour in both positive and negative ways. For example the law is seen as a skilled activity necessary for the smooth functioning of all society. Lawyers outwardly wear uniform (wig and gown) as symbols of expertise and authority. The education of lawyers is based in high entry standards and closed entry into the profession. The state could regulate this entry and open it up but does not generally interfere with this process. Pay is often linked to judgements about value but also reflects professional power to regulate pay and reward. Society may take the view that the occupation needs long educational provision or that it provides an essential service, or both. However, this is not self evident. Why would a professional footballer earn more than a registered nurse—what does this say about the value of care as opposed to the value of entertainment, or does this reflect the relative power of the two occupational groups?

Activity 3.7: Critical thinking (page 71)

You may well find these values in the NMC *Code*, or see the Royal College of Nursing's 'Defining Nursing', available online at ww.rcn.org.uk.

Activity 3.8: Evidence-based practice and research (pages 71–2)

This could really be expanded and argued over!

- It may be suggested that nursing philosophy emphasises the bio-psycho-social elements of human experience while new age philosophy places the human in the same context. Both may see that health has to address all of these elements.
- Both address health and illness but 'new agers' may see medicine as limited in its approach.
- Both centre on health and illness, both use scientific approaches, both place the individual at the heart of practice.

Knowledge review

Now that you've worked through the chapter, how would you rate your knowledge of the following topics?

	Good	Adequate	Poor
1. Structure and process.			
2. Culture and occupational socialisation.			
3. Professional and social identity.			
4. Norms, values, beliefs, attitudes and cognitive dissonance.			
5. Occupational socialisation.			

Where you are not confident in your knowledge of a topic, what will you do next?

Further reading

Day, J (2006) *Interprofessional Working.* Cheltenham: Nelson Thornes, especially Chapter 2.

Hornby, S and Atkins, J (2000) *Collaborative Care: Interprofessional, interagency and interpersonal,* 2nd edition. Oxford: Blackwell Science.

Øvreteit, J, Mathias, P and Thompson, T (eds) (1997) *Interprofessional Working for Health and Social Care.* London: Macmillan.

Useful websites

www.spring.org.uk   The home of PsyBlog – a resource for psychology and concepts such as social identity theory.

Chapter 4

Interprofessional working: the doctor–nurse relationship and collaborative practice

Draft Essential Skills Clusters continued

By first progression point:

ii. Works within limitations of the role and recognises own level of competence.

iv. Shows respect for others.

v. Is able to engage with people and build caring professional relationships.

By entry to the register:

xiv. Uses professional support structures to develop self awareness, challenge own prejudices and enable professional relationships, so that care is delivered without compromise.

Cluster: Organisational aspects of care

10. People can trust the newly registered graduate nurse to deliver nursing interventions and evaluate their effectiveness against the agreed assessment and care plan.

By entry to the register:

x. Reviews and makes adjustments to the care plan with the person and in response to evaluation, communicating these changes to colleagues.

14. People can trust the newly registered graduate nurse to be autonomous and confident as a member of the multi-disciplinary or multi-agency team and to inspire confidence in others.

By first progression point:

ii. Supports and assists others appropriately.

iii. Values others' roles and responsibilities within the team and interacts appropriately.

iv. Reflects on own practice and discusses issues with other members of the team to enhance learning.

v. Communicates with colleagues verbally, face-to-face and by telephone, and in writing and electronically in a way that the meaning is clear, and checks that the communication has been fully understood.

By entry to the register:

vi. Actively consults and explores solutions and ideas with others to enhance care.

vii. Challenges the practice of self and others across the multi-professional team.

viii. Takes effective role within the team adopting the leadership role when appropriate.

x. Works inter-professionally and autonomously as a means of achieving optimum outcomes for people.

Chapter aims

After reading this chapter you will be able to:

- understand decision making and professional communication;
- understand the working relationship between professional groups;
- recognise the barriers to collaborative working;
- suggest ways of working positively with other professions.

Introduction

It is obvious that what I have done could not have been done had I not worked with the medical authorities and not in rivalry with them.
(Florence Nightingale in Woodham Smith, 1952)

As we have already noted in Chapter 2, developments in the NHS and government policy have placed interprofessional and collaborative working high on the agenda and have encouraged a more team-based approach to the delivery of healthcare (DH, 1998c, 2000a, b). We saw in Chapter 3 that the three important elements of structure, process and culture have to be considered for successful collaborative working between professionals. Of especial note is the relationship between doctors and nurses.

Research and anecdotal evidence in acute hospital settings indicates that this may be a problem. There are suggestions that hierarchical teams in terms of decision making still exist, challenging the achievement of a modern workforce characterised by equality of status, esteem and formal decision-making power (Salvage and Smith, 2000). However, two trials and a systematic review investigating joint nurse–doctor ward rounds (Jitapunkul et al., 1995; Curley et al., 1998; Zwarenstein and Bryant, 2000) suggest that working together closely may be worthwhile. However, Zwarenstein and Reeves (2000) conclude that this is not enough evidence to glibly conclude that collaboration works.

This chapter will examine some of the evidence that is emerging about the way nurses and doctors work together. The acute hospital setting will be used as a starting point as much of the research is in this setting. The evidence from primary care settings (see, for example, Speed and Luker, 2006) and with other professionals' needs collecting in order to come to stronger conclusions. The relationship between mental health workers and other professional groups is also poorly researched.

The theory underpinning this approach is that professionals are human beings and are open to biases and prejudices that affect all human relationships to one degree or another. Behaviour is also affected by our external context and our internal psychology. Therefore, working relationships will be affected by a range of factors:

- the history of how professions have developed;
- the working context (e.g. hospital, GP practice, military or civilian, critical care, palliative care, continuing care);
- gender roles and socialisation;
- new, developing and extensions of roles;
- individual personalities;
- the educational experiences of professional groups – their knowledge base;
- professional cultures;
- structural changes in the NHS.

Decision making

A key indicator of collaborative practice is decision making within the nature of the doctor–nurse relationship. If groups of people are working together in a way that is based on equality of esteem, power and status, it could be suggested that decision making will not be based on traditional hierarchical roles (and not on mere custom and practice). The principles involved in successful teamworking will be examined in the next chapter. For now, let us accept that team members bring different skills knowledge and insight into any scenario. Theoretically, the team performance will be enhanced if team members are part of the process of taking decisions rather than as mere operators of other people's decisions. This notion, however, needs further argument.

Evidence-based practice and research

When you are in clinical practice, find out who are the important decision makers for such things as referral to services, discharge, treatment options and review. Try to discover why the individuals have that decision-making power. Is there a legal basis for it, for example?

A brief outline answer is given at the end of the chapter.

The social context of decision making in which nurses and medical practitioners operate is dynamic and complex (Svensonn, 1996; Coombs, 2003), which means that professionals often have to take difficult decisions quickly and in changing circumstances. The range of clinical settings (primary care, acute care, mental health, learning disabilities services) and patient conditions is vast and not all of them have straightforward answers. The evidence base for a decision may be weak, unknown or inaccessible. In this context it has been suggested that professionals engage in 'heuristic' thinking as a way of simplifying the decision-making process. Into this often complex practice is now thrown the target of working interprofessionally, which some may feel is an added demand. The notion of heuristics is important as it suggests there is a tendency to take short cuts in thinking due to external pressures.

Activity 4.2 *Reflection*

Thinking, understanding and decision making take place in the real world, where there are usually considerable time pressures, and there may rarely be a full range of information available to support a complete appraisal of the problem at hand. Kahneman et al. (1982) popularised the term 'heuristic reasoning' for thinking and decision making that involves *short cuts*. Heuristics (rules of thumb) are short cuts that are used to reduce the need to process large amounts of information.

Thompson (2003) argues that nurses use knowledge from their clinical experience to deal with the uncertainties they face. However, this way of making decisions can result in overconfidence in their own knowledge base, 'being correct after the event' or with the benefit of hindsight. The reliance on clinical experience means that nurses must use short cuts that introduce biases into decision making.

- Is collaborative decision making, by definition, a more complicated process that makes taking short cuts by an individual even more common?
- Identify short cuts in your own thinking – an obvious example from everyday life is driving your car. To what extent do we all stick strictly to the rules of the Highway Code and, in addition, what information do we use when driving along a normal trunk road? Any discussion with an Advanced Motoring instructor about what cues we ought to use when making driving decisions will probably reveal our own short cuts and lack of knowledge. Does this practice apply to nursing?
- Short cuts may be taken because of lack of available information or the need to take a quick decision. Could they also result from needing to fit into a team situation?

Activity 4.2 continued

- Melia's work (as discussed in Chapter 3) suggests that student nurses are socialised into learning nursing. Does this include how to make a decision and the short cuts that more senior staff take?

As this is for your own observation, there is no outline answer at the end of the chapter.

A lack of agreement on the definition and understanding of the term 'interprofessional practice' (see Chapter 1) among nurses and doctors may also be making it difficult to initiate a full examination of whether or not this approach to collaboration in patient treatment actually occurs, whether it improves patient outcomes and whether it generates harmonious teamworking along the way (Leathard, 1994, 2003). Interprofessional working for some may actually mean teams of professional groups working alongside each other but with very little cross-over. For others, it may mean integration and full membership of a larger team. Interprofessional working may be just a new term to describe old practices. The 'handmaiden' days may be long gone, but is the achievement of full partnership in formal clinical decision making more of a wish than reality?

CASE STUDY: THE NURSE AS HANDMAIDEN

The role of the nurse in the past could be seen as that of a handmaiden, there to carry out the doctors' prescriptions with little say in what happened. Doctors have always worked closely with nurses and to argue that doctors gave orders without ever consulting the nurses is overstating the case. However, the nature of the doctor–nurse relationship is still a contentious issue.

Thompson and Stewart (2007) argue:

Both nursing and medicine are noble caring professions with strong traditions, externally characterized by mutual respect and well regarded by the public whom they profess to serve. Although nursing is typically characterized as caring and medicine as curing, both are essentially healing disciplines combining art, science and craft and comprising caring, treatment and curative functions. Thus, there are many more . . . similarities and commonalities than cosmetic differences. However, while the relationship between nursing and medicine should always be cordial and collaborative, tensions continue to simmer beneath the surface of an apparently healthy partnership between the two to serve the wider community. Indeed, the nurse–doctor relationship has often been characterized as strained, even adversarial. Historically, it has been fraught with conflict and divided by professional rivalry; usually because of a real and imagined power imbalance with doctors seen as dominating and coercive.

In the past nurses were educated primarily by doctors and because they were hired by doctors if they were considered to be 'good' nurses, a sex role stereotype of the nurse emerged. The doctor–nurse relationship, often seen as a dominant–subservient one, has traditionally been seen as a man–woman relationship with the latter consigned to a 'handmaiden'

CASE STUDY *continued*

role. Indeed, the relationship has been characterized as the 'doctor–nurse game' – a stereotypical pattern of interaction in which (female) nurses learn to show initiative and offer advice, while appearing to defer passively to the doctor's authority. However, with the increasing numbers of nurses being men and doctors women, this relationship is further evolving, though it appears to be influenced by the doctor's gender.

The reasons for this conflict are many and include the historical legacy of both professions, differences in their educational, training and socialization processes, the sexual division of labor, and overlapping and changing domains and boundaries of practice, especially the efforts of nursing to shed the handmaiden role and assume the role of collaborator and autonomous practitioner.

It has been suggested that the modern professional nurse is now 'above' undertaking traditional care tasks in the quest to become more professional (to lose the handmaiden role) and that this has produced discontent among some medical staff.

A consultant anaesthetist at a London teaching hospital complained of patients arriving for operations with bed sores. On ward rounds, he frequently found himself helping patients to eat. 'The catering staff slam the food down. No one bothers. Spooning food into a patient is just too demeaning for professional nurses, it seems. I always thought nurses were meant to care for patients. I might be wrong. I may have missed the plot somewhere.' Another described the difficulty of trying to find a particular patient on a ward. Every patient is supposed to have his name above the bed. But, in some hospitals, they refuse to display the name 'in case it infringes your autonomy'. He had to translate the nurses' diagnoses. 'They refuse to use hierarchical, male-dominated medical terms, so they will not say the patient is unconscious. No, the patient has to have 'an altered state of awareness'.

The source of the rot is a feminist orthodoxy which says nurses must no longer be the 'handmaidens' of male chauvinist doctors but instead must be their equals. 'Caring', therefore, can have no place any more in nursing since it demeans the nurse. Making sure the very old and incompetent actually eat, or making them comfortable in bed, or helping them wash or dress in a way that maintains their dignity, are all beneath too many modern nurses. Wicked stuff; and nothing short of a collapse in the moral heart of nursing itself.

(Melanie Phillips, www.melaniephillips.com)

The feminist theory to which Phillips refers argues that nurses' subordination (and their service work – Mackay, 1995) centres on class, a marriage-like contract or a patriarchy (Gamarnikow, 1978; Carpenter, 1978; Witz, 1992; Davies, 1995).

Activity 4.3   *Critical thinking, and evidence-based practice and research*

Consider the above extracts. Do you recognise the situations described as having anything in common with the places in which you have worked?

What evidence is there in current clinical practice that the handmaiden role is a thing of the past?

As this is for your own observation, there is no outline answer at the end of the chapter.

The following studies will examine evidence from the UK and elsewhere on nurses' perceptions of the existence or otherwise of interprofessional formal decision making among doctors and nurses working in acute services and the nature of their working relationships. At the outset we must acknowledge that the different cultural and working practices in other countries may make direct comparison across countries difficult if not impossible. However, discussion of data from such international research is included to demonstrate the point that the question of how to achieve true interprofessional practice appears to be a matter for debate not just in Britain, but also in other developed states.

The influence of the traditional doctor–nurse hierarchy

The literature on doctor–nurse relationships describes a complicated and ever-changing pattern of professional working and this includes the idea that a significant source of stress for nurses is conflict with doctors (Tabak and Orit, 2007). Not only does this suggest ways in which professionals negotiate their own practice in relation to each other, it also implies impacts on the care that patients receive (see, for example, Sleutel, 2000), and as such could be a factor in limiting or enhancing a patient's or nurses' autonomy (Goodman, 2002, 2004).

Stein (1967) discussed the 'doctor–nurse' game, where the cardinal rule is that open disagreement is to be avoided at all costs, and where the relationship between the two parties is carefully managed to ensure that the hierarchy that privileges the doctor's authority is not openly challenged. This study found that nurses would often take decisions, but would frame them in a passive way to maintain the doctors' sense of professionalism. This game would be played out within the traditional 'handmaiden' context of nursing practice. Other texts on the subject examining medical-nursing roles include the work of Etzioni (1969), Freidson (1970), Walby et al. (1994), Hughes (1988) and Oakley (1995), who emphasised the existence of a hierarchical (*patriarchal*) negotiated order. Oakley thus overtly introduces the gender element. Simply put, doctors give orders not just because they are doctors but because they are male.

Concept summary: Patriarchy

The word 'patriarchy' comes from two Greek words – *patēr* (πατήρ, father) and *archē* (αρχή, rule). It describes the structuring of a society on the basis of the family. Traditional families pass on lineage through fathers. On this basis the father is considered to have primary responsibility for the welfare of the family. The concept of *patriarchy* is now often used to refer to the expectation that men take

---

primary responsibility for the structuring of society, acting as representatives through public office. There is a hierarchy in the family and thus in society.

Patriarchy is seen as an ideological system that has come to be defined as a form of male dominance. More specifically, it is an ideological structuring of society whereby certain members of society (men) believe themselves to be in positions of dominance over others (see Simone de Beauvoir (1949) *The Second Sex* and Germaine Greer (1970) *The Female Eunuch*).

Tyke (2004), a practice nurse, states:

I have often wondered why men choose to specialise in gynaecology. A rather outspoken friend theorises that they have to be either perverts or women haters. Misogyny has always run rife in medicine, says she, because of a patriarchal society that suppressed women. Physicians were traditionally men with power and status (not much change there, then). Women, when not keeping house and churning out offspring, did the grotty jobs like cleaning, laying out the dead, and, of course, nursing.

Today I saw nine women in morning surgery, all harping on about fairly nebulous symptoms. There was nothing to get your teeth into and actually treat, like good old conjunctivitis or an ingrowing toenail. At a bit of a loss, it was all too convenient to cop out: 'It's your hormones, luv, we're all slaves to them'. And this excuse was stoically accepted.

My busy, practical side wanted to deal with these patients sharpish and get on, but my feminist side was ashamed at trivialising their complaints. For, as my friend points out, demanding women are easily dismissed as hormonal.

Medical statistics show that women make up the vast majority of patients attending general practice. So are women a bunch of hypochondriacs with too much time on our hands?

The Ancient Greeks blamed everything on the uncontrollable, wandering womb and then that crackpot Freud came along and diagnosed all women as hysterical. Women probably do come to surgery more than men, but not necessarily because they are ill. They frequently consult for health-related matters, like contraception or smears. Often they are the only adult who is available to accompany a child, so indeed we do see many female customers in this job.

If unwell, women often request female doctors. Perhaps they expect them to naturally be more empathetic, especially with matters 'down below'. Not necessarily so. A female GP I know totally rejects the possibility of PMS, considers post-natal depression to be the punishment of wimps and generally hates seeing women patients. Mind you, she rather fancies herself as a bit of a babe and flirts with anything sporting a Y chromosome. The male patients, of course, lap it up.

In this piece there are a few comments that need further analysis. If women make up the majority of patients in GP practice, what are the real reasons? Do certain conditions fall into 'legitimate' and 'non-legitimate' medical concerns, and who decides this (note the debate around ME)? Are these decisions purely based on medical science? Does culture play a part?

It is suggested in other literature that the traditional hierarchical nature of medical and nursing roles no longer exists, or is at least far more complex than the simple 'handmaiden' model described (Hughes, 1988; Svensonn, 1996; Allen, 1997; Snelgrove and Hughes, 2000). Even so, Martin (1998) argues that this does not mean that hierarchies have completely disappeared as nurses continue to be subject to, as well as creators of, hierarchical structures in many organisations.

Zelek and Phillips (2003) argue that there is *limited research on interactions between female nurses and doctors*, but they go on to suggest that it is the influence of gender that is more important than hierarchical professional boundaries. They cite Glenn et al. (1997), arguing that nurses experience greater satisfaction when communicating with female medical staff and that they prefer a more 'female' managerial style (see Baird and Bradley, 1979; Camden and Kennedy, 1986, but both are dated studies). However, there is the suggestion that female doctors may have difficulties with respect (Tannen, 1994), are under more scrutiny (Firth-Cozens, 1990) and experience unequal treatment from nurses (Pringle, 1996, 1998).

Rothstein and Hannum (2007) undertook a small study in the United States and argue:

Relationships between registered nurses and physicians have often been described in terms of two models: one based on interactions between two health professions and one based on the patriarchy of male physicians and the deference of female nurses.

To evaluate nurses' perceptions of the two models, 125 advanced practice nurses at a statewide professional conference completed a closed-ended self-administered questionnaire that asked about their relations with male and female physicians. Nurses rated male and female physicians very similarly; both groups were rated most favorably on their confidence in the nurse's expertise and least favorably on their recognition of the nurse's responsibilities unrelated to the care of individual patients. Nurses rated female physicians under the age of 50 more favorably than older female physicians and rated male physicians of all ages similarly.

These findings provide greater support for the professional than for the gender model of nurse–physician relations.

(p235)

As noted, the context in which doctors and nurses operate may be an important factor in how they work together. The military is an under-researched area and provides an alternative context to that in the NHS. Ebbs and Timmons (2007) undertook a small qualitative study in which they interviewed six nurses and five anaesthetists from a Royal Air Force Critical Care Air Support Team (CCAST). They concluded that 'personality' is a significant factor in the relationship and has been under-analysed in other studies. The study participants all carried military rank and the peculiar nature of that working environment may mean that the individual's personality rather than their gender or professional status was more influential in how they worked together. Despite it being a small study, it illustrates that we may need to look beyond explanations of gender and traditional roles to explain how staff will work together in the future, especially as the NHS context is changing.

Porter (1991) used participant observation to study doctor–nurse interaction in an intensive care unit and a medical ward. Four models of interaction were 'tested' (see Figure 4.1).

The most common interaction found was model 3, 'Informal overt decision making'. Models 1, 2 and 4 were rarely seen. This suggests a departure from Stein's doctor–nurse game, but not full partnership in decision making in a formal sense. As this study is now over 13 years old and was small scale, further research is needed to establish whether model 4 in the current 'interprofessional era' is any more common. If inter-

Figure 4.1: Porter's interaction models.

1. Unproblematic subordination: nurses' unquestioning obedience.	2. Informal covert decision making: the doctor–nurse game.
3. Informal overt decision making: open involvement of some/all nurses.	4. Formal overt decision making: including the nursing process in decision making.

professionalism is to mean more than just hierarchical teams working closely together, model 4 would need acceptance by the professional groups involved.

At around the same time, Stern et al. (1991) studied a paediatric intensive care unit (ICU) and found that nurses were high-frequency information givers but low-frequency decision makers (model 2?), and also suggested that physicians perceived nurses to be of less value to patient care than they themselves were.

Snelgrove and Hughes (2000) interviewed 20 doctors and 39 nurses in South Wales with a view to ascertaining whether Stein's (1967) 'game' was still being played. Stein et al. (1990) had suggested that nurses had stopped playing this game. Their results indicate that although roles were still seen in largely traditional terms, there was some blurring of boundaries. Work pressure, night working and specialist clinical areas (e.g. CCU) particularly affected role patterns, allowing the cross-over of nursing into traditional medical territory. There was a general reluctance by nurses to challenge the doctors' authority but when it was, the concept of patient advocacy was invoked as a legitimate way of doing so.

This suggests that a nurse would challenge a treatment option not by invoking better/different scientific knowledge, or their own status (which would not be seen as equal); the challenge to be accepted as non-threatening would have to be worded in such a way as to make it based on patient preference and choice, i.e. what the patient would have done if they had the power to express their wishes. Nursing advocacy is seen, then, as a legitimate (and safer?) way to express difference of opinion.

The two professional groups in this study legitimised departures from traditional roles in different ways. The doctors emphasised 'on the job' experience for nurses that would make up for a lack of medical education, while the nurses would emphasise education and training, claiming rights to decision making based on their educational preparation.

Mrayyan (2004) used the internet to collect data from the United States, Canada and the UK; 317 hospital nurses participated. This research suggested three factors that enhanced nurses' autonomy in decision making: supportive management, education and experience, while three factors that decreased nurses' autonomy were autocratic management, the *relationship with doctors* and workload. Again, this appears to support the idea that professional identity and/or male/female hierarchies may work against closer collaboration.

Hall (2004), a senior sister in a UK ICU, illustrates Mrayyan's point in recalling that, before her attendance on a leadership course:

> *Nurses tend to accept things rather than challenge them . . . I did not have the courage to alter aspects of care that I was unhappy with . . . I would not fight my corner.*
>
> (p18)

It is not clear from her quote who needed challenging – senior nurses, managers or doctors – and therefore it is impossible to state that this is an example of the 'doctor–nurse' game. However, it is an expression of the submissive culture in which nurses *still kowtow to the medics* (Curtis, 2004, p6) that many nurses may recognise.

Brand (2006) in an ethnographic study examining nurses' roles in discharge decision making in an adult high-dependency unit investigated the roles that nurses take in the discharge decision-making process. One of the findings was that nurses took a submissive role in order to avoid conflict, but this also enabled them to 'manipulate' doctors. This suggests that a playing of the game is still in evidence.

Idealised work roles as a barrier to partnership working

Adamson et al. (1995) surveyed 133 Australian nurses and 108 UK nurses and asked them to rank their own levels of professional satisfaction and that of doctors. They found that the nurses were more dissatisfied with their professional status than doctors were. The UK nurses also perceived doctors to be lacking in their training to deal with the psycho-social needs of patients, and said that the doctors valued the potential contribution of their own profession over that of others. Their conclusion was that medical dominance was a barrier to nurse workplace satisfaction. This in turn may impact negatively on the decisions nurses are able or willing to make regarding a patient's wishes.

Davies (2000) similarly argues that gender issues that support old ideas of professional working are unhelpful; it is time for old 'doctor' and 'nurse' stereotypes to go.

Sweet and Norman (1995) undertook a selective literature review of the nurse–doctor relationship. They concluded that, while much has been written generating anecdote and opinion, there had been little empirical work to establish an evidence base around the impact of patriarchy on this relationship. They cite some empirical work – e.g. Heenan (1991) and Mackay (1993) – that suggested dissatisfaction and poor working relationships among nurses, resulting in negative consequences for patients. However, much of this research is over ten years old. They argue that the relationship is characterised by each profession having ideal expectations of each other that are not always met. The hospital setting and clinical speciality may also impact on how doctors and nurses work together. They also suggest that further research would benefit both parties in the attempt to highlight strategies that reduce the potential conflict inherent in the relationship.

Rosenstein (2002) reports on the results of a survey in the United States. The first 1,200 responses from nurses, physicians and hospital executives suggest that doctor–nurse interactions influenced morale, and that disruptive physician behaviour (as found in other studies) is a significant stressor.

Chase (1995) undertook an ethnographic study, interviewing ten nurses, and engaging in participant observation in a cardiac surgery unit with 59 nurses and two surgical teams over a two-year period in a US hospital. This study is useful in its suggestion of the notion of two 'parallel hierarchies' of doctors and nurses interacting in a complex manner, and the recommendation that more research is needed on how social contexts affect decision making, and most especially in terms of the place of the patient in this process. Since then, more reports (see above: Snelgrove and Hughes, 2000; Mrayyan, 2004; Hall, 2004; Brand, 2006) have described a hierarchical if not outright patriarchal relationship.

Conflicts in decision making in critical care settings

Sundin-Huard (2001), in a discussion of 'subject positions theory', argues that *'doctors and nurses do not usually take a collaborative approach to the ethical challenges of the critical care environment'* (p376). The result is stress and burnout (as suggested by Sawatzky, 1996). A case study in the UK, describing the interaction between a nurse and a doctor over the care of a baby, is used to elucidate the power dynamic, mutual expectations and discourses available to each individual, and clearly demonstrates how the nurse was forced, in this instance, into a passive role. This suggests that nurses continue to have difficulties in making autonomous decisions and/or have problems with their relationships with medical staff.

The nature of the relationship also may have implications for patients' outcomes. Baggs et al. (1999) reported an association between poor collaboration and poor patient outcomes in three New York ICUs. A patient outcome is the defined end point of the care episode (discharge, death, transfer) or a defined patient condition(s) – e.g. lack of infection, wound healing or stabilisation of symptoms. In critical care, for example, an outcome may be weaning from artificial respiration using a mechanical ventilator. Conflicts and poor communication within care teams may delay a patient being weaned from this machine.

Manias and Street (2001) used an ethnographic approach with six nurses in a critical care unit in Australia. They found that nurses experienced difficulties in decision-making activities during rounds, and that, in addition to not waiting for nurses to join actual discussions, the doctors made nurses feel their contribution was not valued. The key players in this setting were not the nurses but the consultants, who regulated the communication and demonstrated their authoritative positions.

Bucknall and Thomas (1995) surveyed 230 Australian critical care nurses and reported widely varying levels of involvement in key decision making, suggesting that there is particular potential for conflict and role overlap in the critical care setting due to the physical and cognitive closeness of the nursing and medical spheres of work. In a subsequent 1997 study they found that nurses' major sources of dissatisfaction included treatment decisions for patients with poor prognosis and disharmony with medical staff concerning autonomy issues (especially with junior doctors). They also cited earlier research by Bourbonnais and Baumann (1985), in which nurse–physician relationships and prolongation of life were two stress factors (among others) found to be significant hindrances to decision making in the critical care environment.

Sawatzky (1996) described stressful work experiences in critical care in two Canadian hospitals. Ninety-six nurses took part in the study, which used the Critical Care Nursing Stress Scale and the Perceived Stress Scale. Ranking the stress factors revealed that patient care-related issues appeared to be common. The top six factors were ranked for frequency, intensity, threat and challenge. 'Unnecessary prolongation of life' ranked the highest of all, and scored highly in three of the categories. One possible reason for this is that this area of decision making was perceived to be almost completely under the control of physicians. Apathetic, incompetent medical staff also ranked highly in the categories of threat and intensity. These findings, Sawatzky argues, reflect the need to engage in more positive, collegial relationships with medical colleagues. The study paints a complex picture of stressors in critical care, and one that suggests, in common with some of the other studies cited above, that nurse–doctor relationships have to be understood in a complex multi-contextual way rather than as an uncomplicated binary. In other words, it is not just about male–female, doctor–nurse. Other factors play a part, including the working context.

It could be suggested that other factors alluded to in Bucknall and Thomas's (1995) work, and that relate to the theory of social/professional identity (see Chapter 3), are a shared knowledge base and thus a shared professional language leading to shared identity. If groups identify (and value) themselves through various means (including using a particular language), it could be argued that, in certain care settings (critical care) where medical and nursing knowledge overlap (and the language becomes commonly understood and used), there may be a basis for respect and value between the professions. This may operate against traditional hierarchies and patriarchal attitudes. The further apart the knowledge base and the language are, the further apart the profession may become. Of course, it is impossible to identify in any one care setting what the most important factor is, but speaking the right language based on shared knowledge may well be a key aspect.

The stethoscope as a professional badge

The stethoscope is a humble medical instrument that has been used in clinical practice for many years. It may not be just a practical tool. It may also mark one out as a member of an elite profession. Just as judges and barristers wear wigs and gowns to mark themselves out in court as members of the legal profession (why don't solicitors wear this outfit?), medical practitioners may use the stethoscope as a badge indicating their status to others. It could be argued that wearing the stethoscope around the neck is purely practical, as it needs to be to hand, and therefore has nothing to do with status, which of course has merit.

Activity 4.4   *Reflection, and evidence-based practice and research*

Note who wears a stethoscope and when they wear it. Look at images of medical staff in the media. How often are they using a stethoscope as a badge? Note also that the closer to a medical role the nurse becomes, the more likely it is that the stethoscope will be used as an image, especially when theatre 'blues/greens' are worn.

As nurses take on more medical roles (and also when roles overlap in critical care) do they take to 'wearing' the same badge? What message is being sent out?

As the results are based on your own observations, there is no outline answer at the end of the chapter.

Another context is that of palliative care. Martin (1998) suggests that dying people are one group that still had decisions made for them, and quotes several studies that painted a bleak picture in relation to patients' ability to make choices. He suggested, however, that the palliative care movement and hospice care is bringing about changes to the previous status quo. His study highlights the influence of power relations on interpersonal relationships, including those with the patients, and he argues the need to analyse both the power that nurses exercise, and that which is exercised upon them.

A key context relates to decision making about the possible withdrawal of treatment altogether. Goodman (2002) suggests that the Ms B case (refusal by a Trust to withdraw treatment) indicates a lack of a nursing voice in the decision-making process, despite ICU nurses often being seen as advocates for a patient's wishes. The case may indicate that Porter's (1991) model 4, 'Formal overt decision making' (see page 94) was absent in this case, as the court transcript reports evidence and argument from doctors only. This assertion is backed by Coombs and Ersser (2004), who conducted an ethnographic study in the UK in three general intensive care units to study nurse decision making. They concluded that nursing decision making remained undervalued and unacknowledged, despite paradoxically being seen as a vital part of the process by their medical colleagues. They refer to the concept of medical hegemony, which *render[s] nurses unable to influence substantially the decision making process* (p245).

The effects of role change on nurse–doctor relations

Despite the introduction of changes in policy and practice, there are suggestions that the nurse–physician relationship continues to be problematic in the 'modernising' NHS.

Salvage and Smith (2000) argue that the relationship (based on differences of power, perspective, education, pay, status, class and gender) is in need of:

> reconstruction in a context where sensible debate around roles and relationships is scarce . . . some . . . think medicine is not changing, or only reluctantly, or that change is being imposed from outside by political expediency . . . the core dynamic is the same: nursing . . . is still dancing around the medical maypole.
>
> (p1019)

Douglas (2000) reported a urologist commenting on the notion of 'consultant nurse' as an *insult, a betrayal and a gross misuse of language* (p1085). In the United States, Charatan (1997) reported conflict between doctors and nurse practitioners over their roles and pay in primary care. Spurgeon (1996) reported very similar concerns by doctors about nurses' expanded roles in Alberta, Canada.

In the UK, nurse practitioners (and emergency care practitioners) are taking on (medical) diagnostic assessment, clinical examination and treatment roles in emergency and minor injury/illness care. Medical practitioners, although they have always been involved in educating nurses, are becoming heavily involved in the teaching, assessing and mentoring of nurses in the development of these advanced roles. These new developments need further research to clarify how this is working in practice (see Cooper et al., 2007).

Radcliffe (2000), in discussing the nursing profession's struggle to professionalise and gain equality with doctors, suggests that nursing has missed an opportunity to strengthen its own core values by taking on such things as expanded roles:

> doctors are more than happy to see nurses do tasks that usually take up time and quite frankly bore them (IV drugs, endoscopies, pre op assessments, prescribing). The doctors, however, are still having their needs met by nurses.
>
> (p1085)

This sentiment has been reflected in a recent RCN congress motion regarding the retention of technical tasks for nurses, while caring is devolved to care assistants (Wright, 2004). This comment implies that nurses are still dancing around the 'medical maypole' by 'dumping' care and taking up technical tasks as suggested by Radcliffe.

This proposition is empirically supported by Jones (2003) who reports on the experiences of nurses in acute settings (2 teaching hospitals in the UK, 24 participants in 4 focus groups) and argues that nurses are taking on the technical activities of junior doctors, while care assistants are undertaking nursing tasks. While this is a small study and cannot be generalised (it is also based on reporting so we do not know the actual behaviour), these task and role changes may be an unforeseen product of the shift to interprofessionalism and the blurring of boundaries, which in this context should perhaps mean the redefinition of the nurse as a junior doctor. This in turn could lead to the redefinition of care assistants as nurses.

Primary care

Much of the preceding discussion has been drawn from acute hospitals. This reflects the fact that much of the research is hospital-based. However, we can get an idea of whether similar experiences in the relationship between nurse and doctor exists in GP practices. Speed and Luker (2006) examined the ways in which district nurses and general practitioners interacted and influenced each other's work within primary care services. They used a qualitative approach using data from 300 hours of participant observation and 40 semi-structured interviews with 33 district nurses. They argue:

> *The shift in power to general practitioners (GPs) has meant that they can exercise ever-increasing authority over nurses in their employ. Strict rules governed the process of inter-professional work and nurses and doctors used creative strategies to overcome the problems that existed between them. The data show that nurses could and did resist the power of GPs but this resistance generally elicited other more punishing forms of authority. Direct and indirect threats were commonplace. The data suggest that district nurses were moving into a closer, more business-like and tightly-controlled working relationship with general practitioners.*

Note the use of the phrase 'other *punishing* forms of authority'. This is strong language to describe the relationship.

It has been argued in a previous (much older) study in another primary care setting (MacIntosh and Dingwall, 1978) that the subordination of nursing to medicine and the 'fallacy' of egalitarian teams is based on three factors.

1. Doctors and nurses are trained within a hospital structure at the outset of their careers and in this situation nurses learn their subordinate roles. This then will be carried out in their following careers in primary care. (This is known as socialisation.)
2. GPs have a long history as independent practitioners in the NHS alongside their status as 'contractors' of services, staff and amenities (including the hiring of district nurses). After all, the modern GP practice is a business that places the GP partners also as direct employers of nursing staff.
3. Gender: GPs have tended to be men, while nurses are women.

Activity 4.5   *Critical thinking*

Evidence from primary care is very scarce. The work of Speed and Luker, and Macintosh and Dingwall (though separated by quite some time) suggests a relationship not unrecognised in hospitals. However, these are only two studies, and they both relate primarily to one group of nursing professionals – practice nurses – rather than to all nurses working in community settings. Consider whether they have any merit as descriptions of the relationship.

As this is for your own consideration, there is no outline answer at the end of the chapter.

Mental health care

Students on the mental health nursing programme will share many experiences and characteristics with the adult nursing branch. However, there are some major differences that may affect their working relationship with psychiatrists and clinical psychologists.

- Is there a higher ratio of male to female mental health workers and, if so, does this change the nature of the working relationship with (male) psychiatrists?
- The education and the working environment is not as hospital-based as it is for the adult branch.
- Caring philosophies are transforming into therapeutic interventions that increasingly resemble the work of other therapists (for example, counsellors and psychologists).

Again, context and gender are issues, but how this actually is experienced for mental health practitioners is difficult to judge.

Jones (2006) reported on findings to identify some of the difficulties encountered by the multidisciplinary team in the development and implementation of a care pathway for patients diagnosed with schizophrenia. He argues that the introduction of patient care processes such as *care pathways* are relatively new for psychiatry and will potentially uncover tensions within the team. Data were collected in an acute psychiatric unit:

All clinicians argued strongly for clear role boundaries but also defended their perceived control over health care from other professions. The findings indicate that designing a care pathway for people with schizophrenia may produce conflicting perceptions from the team. Conflict may arise through professions being unwilling to accept plurality over roles, which may hinder progress in meeting the needs of patients. The findings also counter the impression that care pathways can be implemented with little impact on the team.

There is no suggestion here that gender is the issue; rather, it is the need to collaborate and develop a care pathway that has opened up potential differences of view.

Brimblecombe (2005), in an attempt to study the relationship between mental health nurses and psychiatrists within the UK, argued that:

psychiatry emerged as a profession at the end of the 18th century and found a power base within county asylums from the middle of the 19th century. Medical superintendents, the doctors in charge of asylums, had strict control over the activities of attendants, the justification for which was the need to protect patients from cruelty and neglect. Superintendents' desire for their own enhanced professional status led to formalized training for attendants at the end of the 19th century, in which training materials again reinforced the importance of obedience by nurses (as attendants had become known). During the 1920s, trade unions struggled for improved pay and conditions, whilst professionalizing mental health nursing was a secondary priority. Reorganization following creation of the National Health Service in 1948 lessened super-intendents' authority, and ultimately the management of mental health nursing shifted from them. The move towards community care allowed mental health nurses to develop greater independence, which was supported by changes in nurse education.

However, he concludes:

Psychiatrists in the UK remain highly influential, despite the move from their traditional power base in hospitals. Changes in mental health care, such as new nurse prescribing powers and the loss of psychiatrists' control over admission of patients to hospital, will continue to change the relationship between mental health nursing and psychiatry.

The nature of the relationship between mental health nurses and other professions needs continuing research to establish the nature of collaboration, conflict and the impact on patient outcomes. The same applies to learning disabilities nurses.

> **Concept summary: The doctor–doctor relationship**
>
> *The doctor–patient relationship is often spoken about and is typically characterized by one of trust and compassion. However, the doctor–doctor relationship is rarely discussed openly as it is too hurtful to reveal the truth. Lack of compassion, competitiveness and even cruelty abounds in the opinion of the author who exemplifies this by some personal anecdotes and is based on 30 years as a physician. Unfortunately the lessons to be learned occur too late for most individuals. Selection of medical graduates may also play an important role in the whole malady.*
>
> (Allen, 2005)

The potential for increased collaboration and improved patient outcomes

Attitudinal issues, such as dealing with conflict, are important aspects of collaborative working. Skjorshammer (2001) interviewed 29 health professionals in a Norwegian hospital and argues that they seem to use three approaches to handling conflict: avoidance, forcing and negotiation, and usually in that order. Avoidance behaviour or suppression is the most common reaction to an emerging conflict. If the use of power (forcing) does not re-establish a balance between the participants, one negotiates. Nurses and physicians in particular seemed to differ considerably in their perceptions of what is a conflict, and when to do something about it.

This latter point is picked up by Coombs (2003), who argues, in a review of literature and a research study, that collaborative working environments had not yet been fully achieved, and that role definitions and power bases within traditional and historical boundaries continue to exist. Three intensive care units took part in an ethnographic study that explored decision making between doctors and nurses:

> *A key issue arising . . . was that whilst the nursing role in intensive care has changed, this has had little impact on how clinical decisions are made. Both medical and nursing staff identified conflict during patient management discussions. However, it is predominantly nurses who seek to redress this conflict area through developing specific behaviours . . . Using this approach to resolve such team issues has grave implications if the government vision of inter-disciplinary team working is to be realised.*
>
> (p125)

Zwarenstein and Reeves (2000) and McCallin (2001) argue that *there is little empirical evidence to suggest that interdisciplinary teams improve patient outcomes* (McCallin, 2001, p419), while noting that the changing context of healthcare organisation and delivery supports collaborative interaction. Concepts of primary nursing, the nursing process and total patient care have affected interprofessional working, as the emphasis has moved towards teamwork. Reviewing the literature on interprofessional working and teamwork, several issues were noted: communication, redefining roles and breaking down stereotypes early in professional education were key factors. Many of the studies cited in McCallin's paper were published between 1985 and 1997, with two from 1999 (New Zealand), and therefore there is a need to study clinical teams and educational processes as they operate in the twenty-first century.

McCallin concludes that interprofessional relationships have been studied without linkages to a broader context, the socio-historical backgrounds being notably absent.

The label – be it interprofessional, interdisciplinary, multiprofessional and so on – applied to teamwork in healthcare is unimportant. How teams actually work together, and whether patient outcomes are improved, are the real issues. As McCallin argues:

> more research is needed to provide empirical evidence grounded in practice of the processes which teams use as they work . . . [and it has to be asked] does . . . interdisciplinary practice improve outcome management?

> (p428)

However, McPherson et al. (2001) argue that interprofessional collaboration *has* improved patient outcomes in a range of settings, including primary care. They cite 19 studies that report such outcomes as decreased mortality in stroke patients, coronary artery bypass surgery and traumatic brain injury. These studies were published mainly from 1997 to 2001 (n = 14), in the UK and North America. They argue that the evidence is that *teamwork works* (p47), although they acknowledge that there are methodological difficulties of the research in some of the studies cited. Interestingly, they also state that *an explicit inter-professional approach may not always be needed to achieve the [patient] outcomes* (p47). It may also be noted that they express the view that teamwork may not be the same thing as interprofessional collaboration.

The role of education in encouraging interprofessional working

Will interprofessional practice lead to more collegiate decisions that will improve patient outcomes, and what role should education play in preparing new doctors and nurses for this cooperative way of working? Davies (2000) asks whether there is any collaboration and cooperation between the two professions, and states *there are good reasons why doctors and nurses are not far along this road* (p1021). Davies argues that a medical education that emphasises expertise, autonomy and responsibility more than interdependence, deliberation and dialogue has taught doctors to be self-reliant and independent, while, on the other hand, nursing traditions have emphasised hierarchy and rule following. The submissive emphasis in nursing may have diminished of late, but there is still a weight of traditional thinking (including gendered thinking) that both professions adhere to. Davies concluded that, while education may challenge this emphasis on privileging the view of the independent-minded doctor over that of the more collegiate-thinking nurse, there is still a long way to go.

While maintaining a positive spin on interprofessional education and collaboration, McPherson et al. (2001) recognise some important barriers. Educationally, they point out:

- scheduling challenges – linking programme timetables;
- variations in learners' ages, educational level and clinical experience;
- differences in academic policies between institutions and programmes;
- the complexity of the design for interprofessional education and the considerable time and commitment needed.

In the context of the discussion above, they also point out attitudinal barriers:

- differences in financial reward and professional goals;
- differences in language;
- historic rivalries;
- fear of the dilution of professional identity.

They argue that these attitudinal barriers are pervasive and hard to address, one reason being the experience of clinical practice:

A student who sees competition rather than collaboration among professionals will discount prior classroom based teaching that claims the benefits of inter-professional work.

(p50)

There are other small-scale studies reporting interprofessional education (medical and nursing students working together) that provide tentative evidence for the breaking down of barriers. Collings and Goodman (2003) report a project teaching Advanced Life Support and 'breaking bad news' to both groups, and Cooke et al. (2003) also discuss 'breaking bad news' education. Results indicate that nursing and medical students valued the education provided, and see themselves working more closely together as a result, as well as challenging stereotypes (female nurse – male doctor). However, as Collings and Goodman suggest, there need to be follow-up studies to test the longevity of these results. The following chapter will address the educational issues in more detail.

Conclusion

The research literature underpinning the success of interprofessional practice, especially that of the doctor–nurse collaborative process, is not extensive across all branches of nursing and across all healthcare settings. However, evidence from other countries as well as the UK suggests that, in acute settings, the level equality of esteem and power in formal decision making indicates a continued imbalance in professional roles of doctor and nurse. Whether this negatively impacts on patients' outcomes cannot be stated with any certainty. There appears to be evidence that teamworking may improve outcomes, but teamworking is not necessarily the same as interprofessional collaboration, equality of decision-making powers or status, which 'interprofessionalism' may imply.

While the influence of the traditional doctor–nurse hierarchy on decision making undoubtedly has changed, evidence exists to suggest a continued imbalance of decision-making power in certain key areas. Idealised work roles, which work as a barrier to partnership working, are undergoing restructuring in the context of the reduction of junior doctors' hours and GP out-of-hours cover. These and other effects of structural modernisation (e.g. the advent of nurse practitioners in minor injuries and casualty units) on nurse–doctor relations, reflect the adoption of diagnostic assessment and clinical examination roles by nurses that were once the preserve of the doctor.

There is potential for increased collaboration and the opportunity for empirical demonstration that this leads to improved patient outcomes. The role of education in encouraging interprofessional working is crucial, but overcoming the obstacles to a fully fledged interprofessional curriculum is a continuing challenge.

So what can be done?

If working relationships are affected by such things as:

- the history of how professions have developed;
- the working context (e.g. hospital, GP practice, military or civilian, critical care, palliative care, continuing care) – in other words, the organisational structure;
- gender roles and socialisation;
- new, developing and extensions of roles;
- individual personalities;
- the education experiences of professional groups – their knowledge base;
- professional cultures; and
- structural changes in the NHS;

and if a nurse *feels* subordinate and the student nurse's status as junior places one even lower on a hierarchy, what can be done? The following are some suggestions.

- Learn to accept those things that are not changeable, such as your (lack of) experience to date, your (lack of) skills and knowledge.
- Develop your knowledge base – be thirsty for new knowledge, develop information management and retrieval skills. Expand your knowledge of other professionals' roles.
- Understand that gender roles and patriarchal attitudes can be challenged and are changing.
- Understand that the behaviour of others does not always result from superior knowledge – that they are fallible human beings possibly in need of your understanding!
- Don't accept uncritically others' positioning of you as junior and/or female: talk to your tutors about opportunities to learn some assertiveness skills.
- Learn to articulate clearly the needs of your patients and yourself in language that demonstrates your developing knowledge and abilities.
- Develop your skills and insights of working relationships until you can contribute to discussions and organisation of care work.
- See yourself in positions of power and influence in the years to come – try to get a 'vision' of yourself as 'mover and shaker' promoting interprofessional understanding in the future.
- Value yourself.
- Joining with others for emotional support and understanding in sometimes difficult situations can help.
- Realise that modern nursing work can be frustrating, emotionally draining and exhausting, even without touching a patient.
- Accept that change and challenge will be constant companions.
- Learn about and develop emotional intelligence (Goleman, 1995). See Further Reading and Chapters 5 and 6 for more details.
- Develop active networks of support, debate and challenge of current practice – use new media to assist in this (e.g. web-based social networking).

This list is not complete – you may like to add more.

CHAPTER SUMMARY

This chapter examined in much more detail how the two arguably dominant groups in the NHS have actually worked together. This is to illustrate the tensions and cultural differences that hinder collaborative working. The discussion is drawn from research studies that have tried to uncover how doctors and nurses work together as professional groups. It is drawn largely from the work done in acute hospitals and hence is a biased view. It has to be recognised that we would need to examine other contexts in much more detail, especially as recent policy urges interprofessional practice across the board. This chapter gave clues to things that may underpin future practice and would need to be worked on if professions are to change. There is a suggestion that clinical decision making, i.e. how patient care issues are decided, is subject to various influences (gender, for example), not all of them clinical.

Activities: brief outline answer

Activity 4.1: Evidence-based practice and research (page 87)

You may be a member of a committee, as a student representative, which oversees the running of a degree or diploma programme. This may be chaired by a senior lecturer (possibly the programme leader) and will have other academics and clinical staff as members. In this scenario you are not a full team member of the degree programme but a representative of certain views. You may well think that the important decisions (such as the course content) are decided elsewhere. Those involved with decision making have been tasked with precisely that role. If you feel excluded from taking a decision – for example, on the assessment method of a module – you may feel that students views are not taken seriously (this may also be perception). Exclusions from that decision may be based on judgements about knowledge and about the defined role of the members. Note that how one feels about this process rests on a number of often ill-defined or 'taken for granted' rules. These rules may not be known to everyone in the 'team'.

When you are in clinical practice, find out who are the important decision makers for such things as referral to services, discharge, treatment options and review. Try to discover why the individuals have that decision making power. Is there a legal basis for it, for example?

Knowledge review

Now that you've worked through the chapter, how would you rate your knowledge of the following topics?

	Good	Adequate	Poor
1. The doctor–nurse game.			
2. Interprofessional practice.			
3. Decision making and short cuts.			
4. Patriarchy.			
5. Interprofessional conflict.			
6. Role change.			

Where you are not confident in your knowledge of a topic, what will you do next?

Further reading

Goleman, D (1995) *Emotional Intelligence: Why it can matter more than IQ.* New York and London: Doubleday.

McCray, J (2007) Nursing practice in an interprofessional context, in Hogston, R and Marjoram, B (eds) *Foundations of Nursing Practice*, 3rd edition. Basingstoke: Palgrave Macmillan.

Williamson, G, Jenkinson, T and Proctor-Childs, T (2008) *Nursing in Contemporary Health Care Practice.* Exeter: Learning Matters.

Useful website

www.tandf.co.uk/journals Search for *Journal of Interprofessional Care.*

Chapter 5

Teamwork

Draft Essential Skills Clusters continued

By entry to the register:

iii. Takes responsibility and accountable for delegating care to others.

iv. Prepares, supports and supervises those to whom care has been delegated.

17. People can trust the newly registered graduate nurse to work safely under pressure and maintain patient safety at all times.

By second progression point:

iii. Contributes as a team member.

v. Uses supervision as a means of developing strategies for managing own stress and for working safely and effectively.

Chapter aims

After reading this chapter you will be able to:

- discuss the difference between a group and a team;
- list the characteristics of an effective team;
- understand how teams develop and function;
- discuss the idea of teamworking and collaboration in healthcare.

Introduction

Most teams aren't teams at all but merely collections of individual relationships with the boss. Each individual vying with the others for power, prestige and position.
(Douglas McGregor, 2008)

Chapter 4 examined the research evidence that tries to describe the nature of the relationship between two professional groups. We noted that professional cultures and identities may play a part in this. This chapter focuses on teamworking. It does not explore interprofessional teamwork or collaboration, but concentrates instead on working within nursing teams. We will focus less on the actual characteristics of professional groups and more on the nature of how people, regardless of education or profession, work together in teams. We need to think about what works and what does not and why. We will need to think about what we have to do to become positive in our approach to enhance patient care, improve our working lives, and avoid the worst excesses of stress and burnout.

The NHS is theoretically based on good teamworking. Our examination of the policy initiatives and professional guidance makes that very clear. We have noted that the Nursing and Midwifery Council has specifically stated that nurses and midwives are to work collaboratively with teams and others (and we have previously defined who those 'others' may be).

There are, of course, autonomous practitioners who may work alone on a case-by-case basis. However, even these lone workers will liaise with others on a very regular basis. Therefore, this chapter will explore how people work and what they bring to a team, apart from the obvious professional understanding and knowledge. We will examine the nature of interpersonal relationships and how facilitating teams enhances the working experience. The word 'collaboration' keeps surfacing, so we must be clear as to exactly what this means so we know how to recognise it when it is happening.

Groups and teams

McGregor's statement above alludes to something that many of us may have experienced. A point for reflection is how that statement characterises your current working life. You have already come across the term 'multidisciplinary team' (MDT), which suggests or implies that the various members of that team are more than just a collection (group) of staff who happen to work in the same physical space. The use of the word 'team' in the acronym 'MDT' presupposes, it could be suggested, that NHS work is more than just a collection of individuals. How far does this reflect reality? In Chapter 4 (p94), the concept of 'parallel hierarchies' (Chase, 1995) was mooted as one characteristic of nurse–doctor working partnerships. This may suggest that there are teams within teams.

Activity 5.1 *Critical thinking*

Whether one works in primary care in the community or in the hospital, one is a member of a 'team'; however, this defines team very loosely. Within the clinic, practice or ward 'team' there may be others.

Chase, in a now older study (1995), suggested that there were at least two parallel hierarchies that could describe the working relationship between doctors and nurses. The idea is that each profession ran its own team, with its own 'pecking order', junior deferring to senior. 'Hierarchy' suggests that not only is communication one way, but so also is decision making. There may well be external factors that affect this (e.g. legal accountability for a patient's care may rest ultimately on the consultant in a hospital setting).

The *Compact Oxford English Dictionary* (2005) defines hierarchy as *a system in which people are ranked one above the other according to their status or authority; or a classification of things according to their relative importance* (p476). There is also submission and dominance implied in the use of the word.

* To what extent does Chase's observation still apply?
* Is a hierarchy a naturally a bad thing?

Nancy Kline (author) stated, *Even in a hierarchy, people can be equal as thinkers* (http://encarta.msn.com). This may be true, but what is important is that staff are given the opportunity to voice their thoughts and that the hierarchy gives opportunity for action on those thoughts.

* To what extent does the working environment encourage thinking?

Brief outline answers to the first two questions are given at the end of the chapter. The third question is for your own reflection.

The common factor for many staff members in the NHS is the patient, and it is the needs of the patient that brings people together. However, just because the patient is the focus of our work does not mean that we will become a team or collaborate. McGregor may be suggesting something quite negative about a 'mere' group and, if true, this means that our clinical experience (if it is only a group) must go beyond group membership to become a team.

So, how does a group differ from a team? The question may seem a little 'academic' (so, who cares?), but think for a moment: the two terms may be defining quite different types of activity and levels of involvement.

Here are two definitions of the word 'group':

a number of people (or things) allocated, gathered or classed together.

(Compact OED, p444)

set of people or things: a number of people or things considered together or regarded as belonging together, people with something in common: a number of people sharing something in common such as an interest, belief, or political aim.

(http://encarta.msn.com)

So, what is the core idea in these two definitions of a group? An answer to that lies in considering what they do *not* say. A moment's thought suggests that these definitions are not saying much about the nature of a group, only that it brings people together with perhaps some (maybe ill-defined?) reason. On this basis we are members of many different groups, all of which have various levels of commitment, understanding, goals, purposes and experiences.

Activity 5.2   *Reflection*

Make a list of the groups you belong to. Describe:

- the level of your involvement/membership;
- your level of leadership;
- your emotional commitment;
- your understanding of the group's purpose;
- the clarity of the group's purpose.

Most people (but not everyone) will have experienced being in a family group:

- your involvement could be total (as a young child) or intermittent (as a young adult living away from home);
- your membership is a given by definition; it is your birthright; it is lifelong;
- how you feel about this only you know;
- does the family have a purpose?

Now think of another group. Does any of this feel like a 'team'?

A brief outline answer is given at the end of the chapter.

For our purposes, working with a group implies no interprofessional or multi-disciplinary characteristic as, for example, you may be a small working group of students. Your membership of a group may be accidental or chosen and the experience will be quite varied. You may think of the characteristics of group membership on a continuum, with 'family group' at one end and 'group work' in class at the other.

Activity 5.3   *Reflection*

You will be working within groups already as a student as part of your studies. Sometimes this will be for a very short time period, maybe as part of a teaching session, or for a slightly longer period to produce a group assignment or project. Groups in this sense then are informal, usually with a very defined (hopefully) set objective of completing the course.

Activity 5.3 continued

Identify group work that you have been set as part of your education.

- Identify what worked well and why it did.
- Identify what did not work well and why it did not.
- Did you want to continue working with this group or did the experience make you feel isolated and negative?
- How did you feel about working in this group – was there excitement or boredom?

Think about such factors as:

- the nature of the task you were asked to perform;
- the time limit for that task;
- how well all the group members understood the objective for that task;
- how motivated the group members were to achieve that task;
- the resources the group members had;
- the importance of personality types;
- whether there was a clearly identified leader or facilitator and, if so, who identified this person(s).

As the answers will be based on your own observations, there is no outline answer at the end of the chapter.

It may seem like nit-picking to try to understand the difference between a group and a team, but the point may be to highlight that teams are (should?) be more than just a collection of staff who happen to work for the same employer. Teamworking may mean something quite specific, and effective teamworking may need a little development and understanding.

A group *is*, a team *becomes*. Perhaps that is the difference between the two. Groups may be quite easy to start, but to fashion these collections into teams takes time, energy, knowledge and skill, bearing in mind that some groups, by definition, can never become 'teams'.

Before we leave this notion, let us examine the nature of group working as this is common in both education and practice. A good source of information on this topic is published by the NHS Institute for Innovation and Improvement, which has produced a series of guides on the topics of leadership, management and improving quality (www.institute.nhs.uk).

Activity 5.4   *Reflection*

In *Working with Groups* (www.institute.nhs.uk/improvementguides), the question is posed 'What is an effective group? Suggested responses are:

- the task, objective or the reason for people to meet is well understood by everyone;
- the atmosphere of the group tends to be informal, comfortable and relaxed;
- there is much discussion in which everyone participates;
- everyone listens to each other;
- people are free to express their feelings as well as ideas;

Activity 5.4 continued

- disagreement and criticism are frequent and frank, but the group is comfortable with this and shows no signs of avoiding the conflict;
- decisions are reached by a consensus in which it is clear that everyone is in general agreement;
- when action is taken, clear assignments are made and accepted;
- the leader of the group does not dominate but is in control.

However, a poorly run group or team will:

- be dominated by a few individuals and their perspectives;
- never hear the ideas and comments from the quiet members;
- take too long to get to the real agenda;
- have no clear objectives;
- have no follow up actions.

Following on from your identification of group work that you have participated in, identify from the above what your experience has been.

As the answers will be based on your own observations, there is no outline answer at the end of the chapter.

Reflecting upon what makes a group work you may feel that a key skill is that of the facilitator of the group using what are often known as 'soft skills' or people skills. Look again at Activity 6.4: how many of those points rely on an understanding of people and personalities? It could be argued (assuming that a clear leader/facilitator exists in a group or team) that this person needs to employ skills from the *affective domain* of learning as well as the cognitive. It may be the case that group leaders need *emotional intelligence*, a term that was introduced in Chapter 4, and that will be explored in more

Concept summary: Soft skills

These skills are related to dealing with people, rather than objects, products, processes and ideas, and include:

- communicating;
- team managing;
- influencing;
- encouraging;
- delegating;
- appraising;
- presenting;
- motivating;
- and, in a nursing context, 'caring'.

Thus, 'soft skills' refer to a range of personality characteristics, social graces, language skills, personal habits, friendliness and a positive outlook that people have to varying degrees. Soft skills should complement 'hard skills', which have been described as the 'technical' aspects of the job (your psychomotor and cognitive nursing skills).

Soft skills can be transferable to a wide range of working settings. Development of these skills enhances employability. They may be harder to measure.

detail in the next chapter. At this stage we may acknowledge that the skills needed for group facilitation and leading are similar to those for team leadership. In the healthcare setting, who are the key staff who act as 'facilitators' of groups and teams?

Domains of learning and their application to leading groups and teams

The following three well-known words in the education, business and leadership worlds are known more simply as knowledge, attitudes and skill (KAS).

- **Cognitive**: relating to the intellect (knowledge – thinking).
- **Affective**: relating to feelings, emotion and behaviour (attitude – feeling).
- **Psychomotor**: relating to the manual and the physical (skill – doing).

You may also come across the Knowledge and Skills Framework (KSF) in the NHS, which, at its simplest, is a list of knowledge and skills competencies that staff in the NHS should have. A 'domain' is the academic word used by Bloom (1956) and his colleagues in the development of his 'taxonomy' in *Taxonomy of Educational Objectives: Handbook 1: The cognitive domain* and *Taxonomy of Educational Objectives: Handbook 2: The affective domain*. The third (psychomotor) domain was left for others to develop. See www.businessballs.com for an excellent discussion. A 'taxonomy' simply means 'classification' and 'domain' means 'area of knowledge', or a 'category of knowledge'.

The application here is that facilitation involves not just the ability to think (cognitive) or to have a knowledge base (cognitive) at the appropriate level, but also to be highly skilled in the affective (attitudes, feeling) domain. This means that you will be able in the cognitive domain to store and recall information; understand ideas, arguments and concepts; apply these ideas and thoughts to situations; analyse (break down complicated thoughts and ideas to see what they are made up of and where they come from); and, at the highest level of your development, synthesise (create, build, join) and evaluate (judge the worth or value of).

In the affective domain, the highly skilled will be aware of emotional issues; respond appropriately to, for example, expressions of personal feeling; place appropriate value on ideas and people; and be aware of their own value system.

Facilitating a group requires skills of organisation and sensitivity to others. It should not be confused with:

- chairing a meeting or debate, which is more directive and aimed at particular outcomes and objectives;
- counselling or group therapy, despite having elements of understanding people;
- teaching or training.

Activity 5.5   *Critical thinking*

How may we judge whether a teaching session, a clinical experience or group work has been positive? What measures may we use?

- We could think about the objectives. Have they been met? Have we done what we set out to do?
- In meeting our objectives, what if we felt uneasy, anxious, threatened or pushed?
- What if the objectives have not quite been met but we have a better understanding of ourselves, each other and the issues?

Activity 5.5 continued

Thus, what is important – the product or the process? Your feelings about this may dictate your handling of meetings, teams and groups, and may influence how you measure success. Are you 'goal directed' (meeting the objective, getting the work done is most important) or 'people directed' (meeting staff needs, encouraging, motivating, praising)?

Of course, you may think that this question is a 'false dichotomy' (the setting up of two alternatives as if they are mutually exclusive, when in fact there may be other alternatives).

As the results will be based on your own observations and experience, there is no outline answer at the end of the chapter.

The nature of nursing work and teams

Much of what we have just discussed is in very abstract terms. Your task is to apply this to actual nursing work. Herein lies a problem because nursing work is as varied as the people who are nurses. Just think about all the different settings within which nurses work, the different client and patient groups, and the different sets of skills and knowledge needed. The NMC has described broad sets of competencies to be achieved for nursing students. They are general statements that have to be interpreted in the large number of clinical settings. Therefore, when we discuss such concepts as 'team-working', we may be able to think about what has been described in other non-nursing settings and contexts, but our task is to turn that thinking into applying it to real nursing work situations. For example, you will need to identify when nurses (and others) sit down in groups or teams to work together. In many commercial organisations there are regular meetings of staff to work on projects. In nursing one may have a handover and then work either individually or with a very small 'team'. The handover does not resemble a team meeting at all; it is only an exchange of patient information. We may legitimately ask how many nurses are actually working in teams. To what extent, therefore, do nurses have real collaborative practice?

To begin to pick up on how nurses are organised, we may need first to think about the purpose of a team. Although what follows describes in an ideal and abstract way what a team may be, the usefulness of this approach lies in understanding the factors that are said to improve team performance and hence other outcomes, whether they are productivity, innovation or adaptation to change. Once we understand the key factors, we may be able to put some of them into practice and/or encourage our colleagues to do the same.

A warning, though, as all of this is working with people and working cultures, we must accept that the process could be quite tricky. Also, as a student nurse you may feel that this is not what you entered nursing for. You may even be feeling some cognitive dissonance about this whole project. You may also notice that we are using the language of business. You may think that this has little to do with nursing. Much of team (and leadership and management) theory is drawn from academic work other than from nursing, so the focus has been on commercial organisation and culture. The task is to take ideas and research, apply them to our own context, and ask critical questions of both the theory and our own working environments.

Concept summary: Teamwork – understanding the term

Xyrichis and Ream (2008) undertook a literature search and what is known as a concept analysis to try to understand how the word 'teamwork' was being used and what it meant in the healthcare setting. They conclude:

Teamwork is seen as an important facilitator in delivering quality health-care services internationally. However, research studies of teamwork in healthcare are criticized for lacking a basic conceptual understanding of what this concept represents. A universal definition for healthcare settings and professionals is missing from published literature.

Teamwork is proposed as a dynamic process involving two or more healthcare professionals with complementary backgrounds and skills, sharing common health goals and exercising concerted physical and mental effort in assessing, planning, or evaluating patient care. This is accomplished through interdependent collaboration, open communication and shared decision-making, and generates value-added patient, organizational and staff outcomes.

Praising the value of teamwork without a common understanding of what this concept represents endangers both research into this way of working and its effective utilization in practice. The proposed definition helps reconcile discrepancies between how this concept is understood by nurses and doctors, as well as allied health professionals. A common understanding can facilitate communication in educational, research and clinical settings and is imperative for improving clarity and validity of future research.

A team, then, as already indicated, is more than just a group. We may understand a team to be a group of people who are brought together, or who come together voluntarily, to work together but to do so in a collaborative manner. Collaboration may be a defining characteristic of a team.

Collaboration for a team is about reaching a shared goal or task for which the members hold themselves mutually accountable.

Concept summary: Collaboration/collaborate

The following are some definitions of 'collaboration/collaborate':

- *to work jointly on an activity or project* (Merriam-Webster's Online Dictionary, 2007, www.m-w.com/dictionary/collaborate);
- *to work jointly with others or together especially in an intellectual endeavour* (Encyclopedia Britannica Online, 2007, www.britannica.com);
- *collaboration is the process people with different ways of seeing the world interact to learn from each other in order to get better at what ever they are trying to do* (en.wikipedia.org/wiki/Collaborate);
- *Collaboration is a structured, recursive (repeated) process where two or more people work together toward a common goal – typically an intellectual endeavour that is (may be) creative in nature – by sharing knowledge, learning and building consensus* (http://en.wikipedia.org).

- *Collaboration (may) not require leadership and it is suggested can even bring better results through decentralisation and egalitarianism (http://en.wikipedia.org).*

Team: a definition

*A team is a group of people with a high degree of **interdependence** geared towards the achievement of a **common goal** or completion of a **task** . . . it is not just a group for administrative convenience. A group, by definition, is a number of individuals having some unifying relationship.*

*Team members are deeply **committed** to each other's **personal growth** and **success**. That commitment usually transcends the team. A team outperforms a group and outperforms all reasonable expectations given to its individual members. That is, a team has a **synergistic** effect . . . one plus one equals a lot more than two.*

*Team members not only **cooperate** in all aspects of their tasks and goals, they share in what are traditionally thought of as **management functions**, such as planning, organizing, setting performance goals, assessing the team's performance, developing their own strategies to manage change, and securing their own resources.*

(Clark, 2008)

What key ideas is Clark trying to get across here? Note the following words and phrases:

- interdependence;
- common goal/task;
- commitment to each other;
- personal growth and success;
- synergy;
- cooperation;
- sharing management functions.

To what extent does Clark's description of a team fit nursing work? What is the nature of nursing work and does this assist in developing this sort of team?

- Take any of the factors mentioned by Clark and look for evidence of it in clinical practice. For example, interdependence . . . this means that without a team member the others have difficulty functioning. Do not confuse this necessarily, though, with always having to have a particular person in the role. A team member can be replaced by someone with similar knowledge, attitudes and skill – think of football substitutions (or any other sport). Think carefully about this, because at first glance it seems obvious.
- Identify your working team: describe it in the terms that Clark uses. Describe the professions who you think are core members of your team. On a scale of

Activity 5.6 continued

> 1 to 10, with 1 being 'group' and 10 being 'team', as per Clark's criteria, rate your working 'team'.
> - If you think that there is something missing, something that could be developed, how would you go about it?

The answers to these questions will say as much about you as they will about the working environment.

As the questions are for your own observation and experience, there is no outline answer at the end of the chapter.

To what degree does Clark's understanding overlap that of Xyrichis and Ream (see p113)? Pick up on the same words used.

Clark (2008) goes on to argue three points:

A team has three major benefits for the organization:

1. *It maximizes the organization's human resources. Each member of the team is coached, helped, and led by all the other members of the team. A success or failure is felt by all members, not just the individual. Failures are not blamed on individual members, which gives them the courage to take chances. Successes are felt by every team member, this helps them to set and achieve bigger and better successes. In addition, failure is perceived as a learning lesson.*

We place a great deal of emphasis on mentoring in nursing; the helping, coaching and leading of student nurses is an explicit role for the qualified nurse:

Students on NMC approved pre-registration nursing education programmes, leading to registration on the nurses' part of the register, must be supported and assessed by mentors.

(NMC, 2006)

Here we are being given a template, or a checklist against which we can assess our own and our team's performance in this respect.

The team should:

- coach;
- help;
- support;
- lead each other.

Also note the idea of not blaming individuals for failure (a 'no-blame' culture), to which we shall return. Failure is a lesson. So, how do we deal with drug errors in a team discussion? What about poor aseptic technique that leads to cross-infection or poor use of counselling skills, or inadequate suicide risk assessment?

2. *There are superior outputs against all odds. This is due to the synergistic effect of a team – a team can normally outperform a group of individuals.*

Outputs? Before we can say that our teams outperform a group, we need to identify what our performance is and how we measure it. What is our output and is this applicable to healthcare practices? If you argue that it is not, on what basis do you make this claim? To what degree is this clear in nursing practice? Do we have an output that is measurable? What does *synergy* mean?

> 3. *There is continuous improvement. No one knows the job, tasks, and goals better than the individual team members. To get real change, you need their knowledge, skills, and abilities. When they pull together as a team, they will not be afraid to show what they can do. Personal motives will be pushed to the side to allow the team motive to succeed.*

Improvement? In what and how is it measured? Langley et al. (1992) have produced a model for improvement in healthcare sometimes called the PDSA cycle.

Plan – plan your course of action.
Do – put it into practice.
Study – study the results of your actions.
Act – review action based on the study.

It is based on three questions that all staff can ask themselves and/or their teams when trying to improve practice and before they do anything.

1. What are we trying to accomplish?
2. How will we know a change is an improvement?
3. What changes need to be made that will result in an improvement?

The PDSA cycle is then put into action. For a fuller discussion, see NHSII website leadership guides.

Stages of team development for the student nurse

Tuckman (1965) and then later (1977) developed a model to describe group dynamics and the development of a team. The *forming, storming, norming* and *performing* model, with the later addition, *adjourning* (Tuckman and Jensen, 1977) has become widely used in management theory and team building (see Figure 6.1).

The following stages may vary in length; in some experiences, teams or individual team members may be stuck in a particular phase. As a student nurse you have a very limited time to go through these stages.

CASE STUDY: STAGES IN 'BECOMING' A TEAM

The NHS clinical governance support team publish case studies and learning materials. The following is an example of how a team may begin to develop.

In a primary care trust, clinical governance (CG) was seen as a low priority by frontline staff, few attended CG meetings. At the time questions were being raised about the future structure of primary care – with new boundaries and organisations planned. The local CG Steering Group decided to nominate a team to join the CG development programme to

---

> ## CASE STUDY *continued*
>
> *'jump start' their efforts. The 'team' had not worked together in this way. Getting lost on their first journey to Leicester really broke the ice. After that start – journeys to Leicester became valued opportunities to get to know one another and find ways of working together. The team learned to understand different professional perspectives.*
>
> ### Lessons
> - Use the unexpected to 'break the ice' – to learn about one another and start new relationships.
> - Travelling together – and other 'time out' – can help a team gel more quickly.
> - Remember, good teams don't just happen. You have to work to make them good.
>
> Source: *Case Study: From No One To Everyone. Getting people interested in clinical governance* (www.cgsupport.nhs.uk).

Forming

Effort at this stage is spent on defining your personal goals. You may be confused as to what the group is really for and your role in it. You may well try to size up the personal benefits relative to your personal costs of being a group member. You may well keep your feelings to yourself as you try to understand the personalities, the cliques, the internally understood methods of communication that the established team members use. As a student nurse, this will be a very common experience as you swiftly move between new clinical groups, each time having to adapt to new situations and personalities. Your relatively junior status dictates your lack of influence on team dynamics and methods of working.

You are introduced. You state why you are there and what you hope to accomplish. You cautiously explore the boundaries of acceptable group behaviour. This is a stage of transition from student nurse as an individual to team member status, and of testing your mentor's guidance both formally and informally.

Figure 5.1: The forming, storming, norming and performing model.

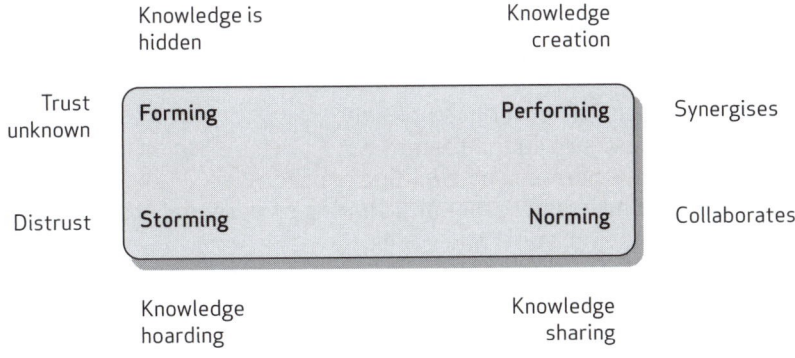

Source: Big Dog's Bowl of Biscuits.

We have found that forming includes the following feelings and behaviours for students:

- excitement, anticipation and optimism;
- getting to know personalities;
- a tentative attachment to the team;
- suspicion and anxiety about the job;
- defining your tasks and role and how they will be accomplished;
- determining the acceptable behaviour for yourself and the group;
- deciding what information needs to be gathered;
- finding out the basics (where do we keep things; where are the lockers?).

Storming

This is the stage when you will be tested. You may well question the values, behaviours, tasks and relative priorities of the goals, as well as who is to be responsible for what. You may well question the guidance and direction of the leader or your mentor/assessor of practice. Be prepared that this stage could be uncomfortable, and you may well feel like withdrawing and isolating yourself either from the emotional tension or because you recognise that your values, beliefs and skills don't fit. If the storming is not allowed to happen, you and the team may never perform well. It is a healthy process in which a team evolves with a common set of values, beliefs and goals. However, the team members must recognise that this is so and encourage the questioning and challenging of accepted norms and values. In your future role as assessor, you may well reflect on this process. Ask yourself whether it is your job to produce a clone or an independent practitioner. If the storming process is protracted, pressure on you will mount and you may feel like leaving. This stage needs careful management and support.

Storming includes the following feelings and behaviours for students:

- resisting tasks and misunderstanding roles;
- resisting changes and suggestions made by others;
- arguing among team members;
- defensiveness, competition and choosing sides;
- questioning the wisdom of those who selected the team;
- disunity, increased tension and jealousy.

Norming

This is when team members' behaviour should progressively develop into an acceptance of differences of opinion that you may bring. Ground rules get established and the decision-making processes are accepted. Your role is understood by yourself and your team colleagues. This is the time when individuals in the group 'value the difference' that others bring. Students in the 'norming' team should feel valued, encouraged and supported.

Norming includes the following feelings and behaviours:

- an ability to express criticism constructively;
- acceptance of membership in the team;
- an attempt to achieve harmony by avoiding conflict;
- friendliness, confiding in each other and sharing of personal problems;
- a sense of team cohesion, spirit and goals;
- establishing and maintaining team ground rules and boundaries.

Performing

Hopefully this stage is reached when the team works effectively and efficiently together and towards the goals. Your goals are accepted as legitimate or have been amended in the light of clinical need. One of your main goals is to have opportunities to learn and to be assessed in practice. This will be a normal part of clinical practice and you effortlessly fit in. The team and individuals learn and develop together.

Performing includes the following feelings and behaviours for students:

- insights into personal and group processes;
- an understanding of each other's strengths and weakness;
- constructive self-change;
- the ability to prevent or work through group problems;
- close attachment to the team.

Adjourning

This is the end of the working life of the team. Some groups such as project teams are created to work with specific problems for a set time – e.g. six months or a year. In healthcare settings, many clinical teams evolve and individual members come and go, but the 'team' stays, never adjourning. If you become a member of a special project team you will experience adjourning. This is not to be confused with the end of your practice placement experience. However, if you have been performing you may feel sad, nostalgic and 'mourn' the end of your experience. We may use the term 'mourning' instead of 'adjourning' as a group prepares to disengage at the end of its lifespan. Student nurses have to experience this process over and over as they move from one placement to another. So it is important for you to recognise those feelings and have support from personal tutors or peer groups as you move from one group to another.

Remember

As a student or future mentor, emotional (affective) experience is just as important as the intellectual (cognitive) experience. You need encouragement to take time out of the process of being in a team, to stand back and ask yourself 'How am I feeling at the moment: angry, frightened, excited, pleased, joyful, friendly?' As a mentor, are you able to facilitate this process?

The above process has been applied to team development but, of course, could apply to the individual joining an established team. The forming and storming process may well be experienced many times throughout your education programme as you encounter new placement experiences.

The matrix team

Often in healthcare you will be a member of an established group or team with a specific task, function or objective, usually defined by the patient or client's needs within a ward or unit. In this context it seems strange to talk about team objectives as the work is to be self-defining. However, you may in the future develop a role as a member of a *matrix team*, or even lead one. Matrix teams may be called different names; these include work groups, task forces, problem-solving teams, committees and special project teams.

Usually, a matrix team is composed of a small number of people from different departments, functions, or organisations who have banded together to solve a common problem or achieve a goal through collaboration. Many organisations have working groups that call themselves teams. The work, however, is produced by a combination of individual contributions, whereas teams produce work that is based on collective effort.

Infection control

Reducing mortality and morbidity from healthcare setting-acquired infection is a key target for the NHS. Nurses will have a role in this.

* Think about how this is being implemented. Is there an infection control team? If so, who are they and how do they operate? What specifically is the nursing contribution to the team? Is evidence-based practice being integrated into the objectives of the team?

Supported living

These services provide support to individuals with special needs, principally adults with a learning disability, in small group living environments or single tenancies. Support is provided based on each individual's needs and ranges from just a few hours a week to up to 24 hours a day. These services enable people to lead a valued life in the community, assisting individuals to make their own decisions and choices and take part in everyday activities.

* If you have had the opportunity to observe this aspect of care, think about the nurse's role in this. Again, identify the team and agencies involved.

As the answers will result from your own observations, there is no outline answer at the end of the chapter.

Factors separating teams from groups

So now we know what stages individuals and teams go through to get to performing, what factors may hinder this process? Don Clark (2008) again outlines some of the major issues that need to be addressed.

Roles and responsibilities

Within a group, and between professional groups, individuals establish a set of behaviours called roles. These roles set expectations governing relationships. In the NHS, when roles begin to overlap in a more formal way, this may be a source of confusion and conflict. Ask yourself what your role is as a student. How might this relate to other health workers – care assistants, for example? Well-functioning teams will have a shared understanding on how to perform their role and perceive the other team members' roles, such as:

* breaking bad news;
* discharging patients;
* reviewing medications;
* choosing appropriate therapies;
* being a patient.

Identity

While teams have an identity, we have noted that professional groups may have their own professional identity; groups may not. A team has a clear understanding about what constitutes the team's mission and why it is important. Members can describe a picture of what the team needs to achieve, and the norms and values that will guide them. If a uni-professional team sees itself as a team apart from the larger group of healthcare staff delivering a service to patients, and in fact identifies itself as such, there may well be little chance that *cohesion* will evolve.

Therefore, to overcome this, open channels of communication at both formal (established and operating in work) and informal level need developing. Chapter 4 noted the challenge in certain settings. It may well be that the working context of many NHS settings do not assist in the development of team identity.

Cohesion

Clark argues:

> *Teams have esprit that shows a sense of bonding and camaraderie. Esprit is the spirit, soul, and state of mind of the team. It is the overall consciousness of the team that a person identifies with and feels a part of. Individuals begin using 'we' rather than 'me'.*

Facilitation

Do you find that discussion at work often gets stuck in seemingly trivial issues or issues that never get solved or addressed? How much time gets wasted in meetings that never go anywhere? A team should use facilitators to keep the team on the right path. Where this is absent there may well be a vacuum that is filled by all sorts of petty jealousies, misunderstandings and lack of 'esprit'.

Communication

This is such an important concept that many nursing texts are written about it. Group members will be centred upon themselves and their individual issues, whereas a team is committed to open communication. You should feel able to state your opinions, thoughts and feelings without fear. Listening is as important as speaking. Conflict is not necessarily negative in a functioning team; managing it positively is the key. Conflict does not necessarily indicate that the team is not working well as differences of opinion are valued. Honest and caring feedback are key to ensuring that members are aware of their strengths and weaknesses. There should be an atmosphere of trust and acceptance, and a sense of community.

Flexibility

Groups may be extremely rigid in how they go about things, sticking to established patterns of work and communication. However, teams maintain a high level of flexibility as they perform different tasks. Leadership is shared among the team. There may well be a formal identified 'leader' but leadership functions do not reside in this one person. In the next chapter we will explore the notion of leadership in more detail.

Morale

Esprit de corps, the spirit of the team, is characterised by positivity – 'can do', 'will do'. You may well feel pride in being a member of the team. When a group changes into a team, members should have the ability to produce results and achieve a high degree of satisfaction in working with one another.

Encouraging great ideas

Creativity, opportunity for innovation and challenge are necessary components to avoid the development of poor practice. The over-reliance on rules and 'custom and practice' stifles creativity. Individuals and teams often become so task-oriented – i.e. 'getting the work done' – that options are closed down. There needs to be adequate investigation of situation and its possibilities.

Activity 5.8   *Reflection*

Reflect on the above factors.

- What practical steps can you take to contribute to the development of a team?
- What skills knowledge and attitudes will you need to develop to become an effective team member?
- What support is available to you and to others to move you forward to become a team?

As the answers will be based on your own observation and experience, there is no outline answer at the end of the chapter.

What sort of teams have you observed while on placement?

Teams are varied in terms of their:

- purpose or mission;
- time they are together;
- the autonomy they have;
- their authority structure.

The *purpose* (mission) may simply be a 'work team' that is concerned with providing a product or a service. In addition, the purpose may be a quality enhancement and *improvement team*. How is your team characterised? Do you see its main function as the provision of healthcare delivery, or can you understand and see its improvement functions? What evidence is there in everyday working that improvement and quality enhancement is part of the process? Ask your mentor.

In most clinical settings, *the time the team is together* is relatively permanent – you will not usually be joining a time-limited team unless it is for a specific project.

Autonomy is harder to gauge. There are formal as well as informal degrees to which team members can make decisions, not just about individual patient care. This is more to do with decisions regarding such things as team objectives, targets, work patterns, education and training, etc. In work groups, team leaders make decisions for team members; in self-managed groups team members have the autonomy to make decisions about their own issues.

The *authority structure* arises from an individual team's speciality or profession. Does the team consist of one profession with a sister or charge nurse acting as a team leader, or does the team have several professions with various professional leaders? The nursing team may have a clear line of authority, i.e. all the nurses take their lead from the sister/charge nurse. The multiprofessional team may have several senior people exercising control over their own profession or other professionals. This may lead to a need to negotiate where the power lies in making decisions.

When you are in clinical practice, try to identify the characteristics of:

- a ward-based hospital team;
- a primary care team.

Compare these in relation to:

- purpose;
- time period;
- autonomy;
- authority structure.

How do the characteristics of the team impact on the experience of working in that team?

As the answers will be based on your own observation and experience, there is no outline answer at the end of the chapter.

Many nurses experience life as member of a *work team*. Initially, you will be working within this type of team. It is sometimes known as a 'production team', i.e. one that performs day-to-day operations – in other words, giving direct patient care.

Work teams may fail for a number of reasons. Many are too interpersonal, others are driven by organisational factors. There may be little trust placed in team members by those charged with leading. In addition, a team may fail due to poor staffing levels and poor skill development and mixture, or working within authoritarian environments. Much may be down to managerial and leadership styles.

Belbin's team role theory

A team role as defined by Dr Meredith Belbin is: *A tendency to behave, contribute and interrelate with others in a particular way* (www.belbin.com/belbin-team-roles.htm).

Belbin's work at Henley Management College identified nine clusters of behaviour, each of which is termed a 'team role'. Each team-role has a combination of strengths and allowable weaknesses. Belbin states that the value of the *team role theory lies in enabling an individual or team to benefit from self-knowledge and adjust according to the demands being made by the external situation.*

The theory is that we may adopt a particular team role and if we go about understanding ourselves and others this allows us to analyse how we work together. Individuals complete a self-test inventory and also get feedback from others to create a profile of the role(s) they may habitually adopt in certain situations.

You will need people with the following roles in any team that wishes to be more than just a production or work team. If nursing work is more than being a 'drone on a production line', if patient care is more than the hands-on (psychomotor) delivery of meeting (highly important), direct patient care needs (the activities of daily living), and includes cognitive and affective elements, there is a need to go beyond the structure of a work team. You will need nurses who are able to fulfil the following nine roles identified by Belbin, which are explained in detail below.

Plant

Do not think of a passive sun-seeking static mind. The plant 'plants' or 'seeds' ideas into the team. They are creative, free thinking, intelligent and may be unorthodox. When faced with the need to innovate or challenge current practice, the plant is a good person to ask. Plants may also be a bit 'geeky' and their personal communication style may be 'different'.

Resource investigator

This is the person you need for pursuing contacts and opportunities. Networking is a key skill here. Enthusiasm at the beginning of the team's work will be directed to contacts outside of the team and they will have information and resource flows from outside. The plant is good at ideas but the resource investigator will acquire them from elsewhere and anywhere. There is a tendency for boredom and a loss of momentum towards the end of a project. The resource investigator is not good at small details.

Coordinator

If not quite the leader as such, the coordinator is the chairperson. This person will step back to see the overview, the big picture. Key skills and attitudes here are confidence, stability, maturity and the ability to recognise abilities in others, and delegation. There is a key role to clarify decisions so that all know what they are supposed to be doing. The downside is that they are seen to delegate rather than 'do'.

Shaper

This is the person who needs challenges and pressure, and will encourage and support others to progress. They may confront head-on obstacles and hindrances. Shapers are the dynamic whip-crackers who provoke their team into action, voicing opinion, saying what others are thinking and encouraging all to do the same in an attempt to push things along. Not necessarily sensitive to the needs and feelings of others in their quest for success, the shaper will 'tell it like it is'.

Monitor evaluator

The monitor evaluators are objective (less emotional?), bringing fairness and logic to an analysis of what is going on. Zen-like in their detachment, they see bias. They are often the ones to see all available options with the greatest clarity. Everything is considered in careful analysis to reach the right decision, which may be too slow for some. However, they can become cynical, curbing enthusiasm for anything that is not based on logic and analysis. Due to a relative distrust of emotion and passion, they may fail to inspire themselves and others.

Teamworker

The teamworker is the 'oil that keeps the machine' running. The key skills of the teamworker are listening, diplomacy, conflict resolution and avoiding confrontation. The oil in the engine is not the most obvious or glamorous part but will be missed if it is not there. Just as an engine becomes noisy when the oil runs out, when the teamworker is absent, arguments may arise. Due to their ability to see both sides and hence perhaps to fence sit, the teamworker may not be able to be decisive when it counts.

Implementer

The implementer is the doer in the organisation, which is a key role. Ideas are turned into action. He or she will be efficient and punctual. Tasks are achieved, often on time. Unfashionable but necessary tasks will be delivered out of loyalty and a sense of team cohesion. On the down-side, getting the implementer to deviate from plans may push him or her out of the comfort zone to appear inflexible and 'bloody-minded'.

Completer finisher

The completer finisher is usually a perfectionist and will often go the extra mile to make sure everything is 'just right'. Tasks and objectives can be left to this person without the need to check, because their own inner high standards drive them towards ensuring completeness and perfection. The completer finisher will not be afraid to check, double-check and then check again, which can cause frustration in other team members who do not share the same perfectionism. They like minor details and may not delegate due to not trusting others to work to their own standards. Valued is a sense of the need for accuracy and they rarely need any encouragement from others.

Specialist

The specialist is the person who has a real passion about their own field of practice and interests. This often means they will have the greatest depth of knowledge and will be on the hunt constantly to improve their knowledge base, so there is little they do not know the answer to. If they do not know they will happily find out. They will bring a high degree of concentration, but only to that specialism. Therefore, they will be uninterested in other aspects of the work. They will enjoy sharing their understanding with others whether it is wanted or not.

Belbin's theory and healthcare teams

What the theory suggests is that in a clinical team, if these various qualities are possessed by individuals, all bases should be covered. If we had the freedom to hand pick a team for a task we might wish this spread of skills. To ensure conflict is reduced and cooperation increased it may be useful to identify the strengths and weakness of team members using this framework in order to celebrate strengths, and predict and understand weakness. It helps to explain why people work in the way that they do. However, beware of stereotyping people in a rigid way; the roles may be in flux and a person may exhibit different roles in different contexts.

A problem with this way of thinking is that it may not take into account the setting within which people work. So, for example, in a clinical area where tasks are clearly described and defined, with particular staff roles assigned to them and with a fixed goal as the 'output', there may be little scope for the plant or resource investigator to flourish, let alone develop in the first place.

Clinical teams cannot choose their team members in this ideal way, unless they are involved with recruitment and selection of team members. Many work autonomously or at least act as lone workers. If Belbin's theory has any validity (truth value) this has implications for how the work is undertaken.

Think of the various patient and client groups (adults and children). These are not abstract tasks to be 'done'. The nature of the interaction that a nurse has to carry out is complex. For example, how will a plant-minded individual fare in a nursing role? Are there some team roles that are better suited to the day-to-day activity of nursing?

Consider the descriptions above. Would you consider yourself as playing one or more roles in teams?

There have been critiques of this typology – e.g. Furnham et al. (1993), Aritzeta et al. (2007). However, Belbin's work is still influential in management training. Fisher et al. (2001) argue that it is more valid to apply the 'Big Five' personality characteristics rather than the nine team roles described above.

- **Extroversion** Desirable traits include characteristics such as excitability, sociability, talkativeness, assertiveness and high amounts of emotional expressiveness. Undesirable traits are introversion, reservation and passivity.
- **Agreeableness** This personality dimension includes desirable attributes such as trust, altruism, kindness, affection and other social behaviours. Undesirable traits are hostility and selfishness.
- **Conscientiousness** This includes high levels of thoughtfulness, with good impulse control and goal-directed behaviours. Those high in conscientiousness tend to be organised and mindful of details. Undesirable traits are carelessness, unreliability and sloppiness.
- **Neuroticism** (emotional stability) Individuals high in this trait tend to experience emotional instability, anxiety, moodiness, irritability and sadness. Undesirable traits are moodiness and being temperamental.
- **Openness/intellect** This trait features characteristics such as imagination and insight, and those high in this trait also tend to have a broad range of interests. Undesirable traits are shallowness and being unsophisticated and imperceptive.

Personality traits as described above are discussed within the discipline of psychology. It is beyond the scope of this chapter to discuss the truth value of this way of looking at how people are. For a fuller discussion see Gross and Kinnison (2007).

Effective healthcare teams

Following a study that attempted to understand the views of a number of healthcare workers, Mickan and Rodger (2005) developed a model that describes an effective healthcare team. They argue that this model can be used by others to understand the important factors that go into making up effective teams. The following factors are suggested in their discussions.

- **Purpose** The study participants described effective teams as *having a well-defined and forward-looking purpose that was relevant to patients and linked with their organisation.* Team members needed to generate the team's purpose to include collective interests and demonstrate shared ownership, both initially and regularly throughout the team's life.
- **Goal** Team goals are links between the team's purpose and its outcomes. Goals are based around the team's task and describe how the team could achieve patient care outcomes. There was a need for team members to agree upon and set goals collaboratively and to describe them in clearly measurable terms.
- **Leadership** This was seen as important for getting the team to achieve its goals. *Good leaders set and maintained structures for making decisions and managed conflict, shared ideas and information, coordinated tasks equally, provided feedback about the team's activity and were able to listen to, support and trust team members.* Study participants also emphasised a need for the team to agree and share leadership functions.
- **Communication** Effective teams have regular patterns of communication where all team members share ideas and information with each other quickly and easily.

There was to be *flexibility of communication patterns to incorporate diversity of team members' interpersonal skills and preferred communication styles.* Clearly written records and sufficient time during meetings to reflect were recommended.

- **Cohesion** *The sense of camaraderie and involvement generated by working together over time.* Through participation in team tasks and consistent communication networks, individuals built up a sense of commitment to the team and trust of other members. Cohesive teams had a unique and identifiable team spirit and individuals shared enjoyment and pride in their achievements. As a result, cohesive teams had greater longevity, because team members wanted to continue working together.
- **Mutual respect** Study participants also described high levels of mutual respect between team members in effective teams, *where individuals were open to the talents and beliefs of each person, in addition to their professional contributions.* As team members accepted their diversity of opinions, they also developed respect for each member's expertise. Mutual respect was also described as a belief that working in a team was the best method for integrating the contributions of all members.

| Activity 5.10 | Evidence-based practice and critical thinking |

1. Team environment.
2. Team structure.
3. Team processes.
4. Individual contribution.

These four categories of the team need to be considered when thinking about what makes a team work. The suggestion is that missing out one of these categories would result in an incomplete understanding. We have already seen in Chapter 3 that 'working together' needs to be based on structure, process and culture. Can you identify a link between the two models?

Six key factors identified by staff in the study were: purpose; goals; leadership; communication; cohesion and mutual respect (Mickan and Rodger, 2005).

When next in clinical practice, see if the six factors are easily identifiable. What would indicate that any one factor exists? Take one factor and look or ask for evidence that it describes the team.

As the answers will be based on your own observation and experience, there is no outline answer at the end of the chapter.

Belbin's team roles describe the individual factors that go into making teams. Mickan and Rodger (2005) have attempted to describe what makes up an effective healthcare team and state that *individual contribution* is one of the four categories of a team. Therefore, there is emphasis in both views that the individual team member should be more than just a 'cog in the machine' if the team is to work effectively.

Willard (1993), working for IBM, identified some key points that should act as warning signs when a team is in trouble:

- members cannot easily describe the team's 'mission';
- any meetings held are formal, stuffy or tense;
- there is a great deal of participation but little accomplishment;
- there is talk but not much communication;

- disagreements are aired in private conversations after the meeting;
- decisions tend to be made by the formal leader with little meaningful involvement of other team members;
- members are not open with each other because trust is low;
- there is confusion or disagreement about roles or work assignments;
- people in other parts of the organisation who are critical of the success of the team are not cooperating;
- the team is overloaded with people who have the same team-player style (see Belbin's roles);
- the team has been in existence for at least three months and has never assessed its functioning.

Activity 5.11   *Critical thinking*

- Are there points in Willard's list that link with Mickan and Rodger's description of an effective team?
- Willard argues that a team is 'in trouble' when 'members cannot easily describe the team's mission'. Does this relate to Mickan and Rodger's factor of 'purpose'?
- How would you know if a team is 'overloaded with people who have the same team-player (Belbin) style'?

As the answers will be based on your own reading, interpretation and experience, there is no outline answer at the end of the chapter.

Teamworking has been seen as generally a 'good thing' but its development is not without problems and difficulties. That is because a 'team' is an abstract idea, but the reality is that you will not be working with an abstract idea. You will be working with very real human beings. Now, in the work setting those human beings will have adopted different identities from who they are at home. They will have been socialised into their professional roles and will have certain values and beliefs that go with that role. However, they have different personalities, dreams, skills, aptitudes and attitudes that they will bring into the working environment. How this blend will actually work out will be the result of a complex web of all these (and more) factors. Your place in it is the most important thing to you, but you will at times feel like a cog in the machine. You will be ignored, or even shouted at. You are special but you may not feel special. At times you will not be treated in a very special way. Therefore, you will need to develop emotional intelligence (EI) as you and your team develop 'team intelligence'.

Activity 5.12   *Critical thinking*

What is the core idea(s) in the following extract, 'Towards team intelligence' (Robbins and Finlay, 2000), Epilogue?

We believe in teams. But teams are trouble, because they're made of people, and people are trouble. The happy-talk books pretended that just murmuring the mantra of teams would cause all the creepy organizational goblins – inefficiency, low productivity, befuddled processes, high cost, bloated workforce, poor morale, poor return on investment – to fall away.

Activity 5.12 continued

Teams would magically outperform the old hierarchical system, and everybody would get along, and you wouldn't need the metal detector at shareholders meetings. Quality without tears.

But hey, guess what – ain't no such thing as quality, or any kind of organizational transformation, without tears. In fact, tears – meaning, sincerity, commitment, and caring about the people you work with – are probably the best sign you'll get that you're on the right track. We talked for so many years about 'the bottom line', meaning quarterly profits, that we have trouble admitting that there are multiple bottom lines to what we do. Besides lying awake at night worrying about return on outlays, team leaders worry about:

- whether leadership is leading;
- whether the team 'gets' the organizational vision, or its own goals;
- whether the full knowledge and intelligence of every team member is being tapped;
- whether the people who make up the team are getting their non-team needs met.

These are not concerns that business schools teach. And yet, in the brave new world of teams that is materializing around us, they are the concerns that will keep the heart of the modern organization pumping blood. Team members don't have to be best friends to be a good team. Every team has people who would not pick one another to affiliate with in a thousand millenniums.

But we're not lovers, or even best friends – we're a team. All we have to do is take one another's side on the main issues – doing the job the team exists to do.

Philosopher Terry Warner talks about a 'principle of agency', by which all team members become agents for one another, charged with the task of making one another's dreams come true.

A better analogy than friends is family. Like members of a family, team members do not generally ask to be thrown together. Like families, all teams are flawed. Like families, teams have their high points and their low points. Fights break out. Emotions flare.

And just as families usually pool together in crisis, and set their misgivings aside, so must teams. After all, we spend as much or more time with team members as we do with our real families. And, the dreams of our real families often are so bound up in the aspirations of the teams we belong to.

In the best teams you see a circle – of sympathy, support, and a limited kind of love. It is the love engendered when team members sincerely want the best for one another.

In good teams, you see at the very least an ongoing curiosity about one another. How can we be so different and still work together? How do we harness the power of our differentness? What must we do to continue to share information and create new knowledge? Curiosity, the key to our intelligence, is the key to team intelligence.

Activity 5.12 continued

If the team movement arose from any single ethic it was that people are not cogs and levers, as the old organizational diagrams suggested. **We are human beings. Ignore the interior workings, the strivings and desires, and team failure is inevitable.** *But when people take the time to learn about one another, what is in their hearts as well as in their minds, we rise to a higher level. Call it love, call it curiosity, call it team intelligence, or don't call it anything at all. But somehow or other, you have to get there. It is the glory of working together, and getting things right.*

An outline answer is given at the end of the chapter.

During the 1970s, a phrase was used in the Royal Navy to describe someone who, though 'bright', lacked a certain skill in practical application. It would be said that they could 'tell you the volume of a jam jar but cannot take the lid off'. This phrase suggests that there is more to intelligence than is usually understood. The principles that underpin the idea of EI argue that the concept of the intelligence quotient (IQ) is only one part of the whole. The EI idea (Goleman, 1995) argues that IQ is too narrow; that there are wider areas of intelligence that influence, shape and direct how successful we are. Success in life and work requires more than IQ (the traditional measure of intelligence), which ignores essential behavioural and character elements. In the next chapter we will be examining in more detail the individual skills, attitudes and ideas that are linked with this concept.

Concept summary: Emotional intelligence and teamworking

Teams are often evaluated for complementary skill mix and expertise that are integrated for specialist service delivery. Interactional skills and emotional intelligence also affect team behaviour and performance. An effective team needs both emotional intelligence and expertise, including technical, clinical, social and interactional skills, so that teamwork becomes greater or lesser than the whole, depending on how well individuals work together. If nursing input into interdisciplinary work is to be maximized, nurse managers might consider the role of emotional intelligence in influencing team effectiveness, the quality of client care, staff retention and job satisfaction.

McCallin and Bamford (2007) argue that high-performing teams need three 'inputs': intellect, expertise and emotional intelligence. The four components of EI – self-awareness, self-management, social awareness and social skills – not only apply to individuals but also to teams.

The role of the nurse manager is emphasised in bringing this to teamworking. To what extent is this a manager's role and what can an individual bring to this understanding?

The learning organisation

Teams operate because of the skills of individuals who make them up. Teams have to operate within organisations. An important factor in how teams are able to work is the structure and culture of the organisation within which they work. It may be fruitful to think about the sort of organisation in which people find themselves. Remember that 'organisation' itself is also an abstract idea that actually alludes to how very real people work together. The rules, cultures, structures and processes that define an organisation are both a product of the people and also produce the people who work in the organisation. People create and are created by their work, and of course some people have more power and influence on how that work will look and feel.

Various attempts have been made to understand how organisations prosper and develop. One writer is Peter Senge (1990), who describes his idea of the 'learning organisation' (LO) as follows:

> organizations where people continually expand their capacity to create the results they truly desire, where new and expansive patterns of thinking are nurtured, where collective aspiration is set free, and where people are continually learning to see the whole together.
>
> (p3)

It may be worth reflecting on some key points here:

- new thinking is nurtured;
- aspiration is set free;
- people are continually learning.

This sounds like an idealised version of the working environment, and it is in response to the idea that only those organisations that can adapt to changes, are flexible in their working and support the talents of the people who work for them will survive in a changing environment. It is the opposite of 'we have always done it this way' thinking.

In the private sector, organisations that do not adapt and change may go out of business. In the public sector there may not be accountability to shareholders and the 'bottom line' but there are pressures for efficiency and effectiveness. The learning organisation can therefore equally apply to the NHS as to Coca-Cola.

Activity 5.13   *Critical thinking*

- Describe the ways in which a clinical setting could be identified as a 'learning organisation'. What would indicate that a clinical area is 'learning' as against one that is stuck in outdated practices?
- Identify key members of staff who could encourage this 'learning'.
- Define what we mean by 'learning'. What is this 'learning about'?

An outline answer is given at the end of the chapter.

The argument runs that people have the ability and willingness to learn, but the structures in which they have to work are often not helpful to reflection and learning activity. Staff may not have the ideas or the guidance to understand and challenge the situations they face. This may result in issues overwhelming workplaces, leaving staff unable to think through solutions. A learning organisation that can harness people's innate drive to innovate and create may be better placed to predict and deal with issues.

Peter Senge argues that learning is core to what it is to be human, but it applies to both individuals *and* organisations. An LO involves what he calls 'generative learning' – learning that enhances the capacity to create. He suggests that, in addition to this, we must understand that people are able to work upon the structures and systems of which they are a part. This understanding of staff in the workplace grasps the point that people should not just be *reactors* to the current working experience; they should have an active role in creating how the organisation progresses.

If the last point is true, we may need to reflect on the extent to which current workplaces encourage both learning and creative activity by both individuals and the organisation itself. Thus, what structures, processes and cultures nurture learning?

Further, we must consider whether nurses have been given the responsibility for change and progress, but no power to put in place structures and processes to affect that change.

If the health service is a learning organisation or is to become a learning organ-isation, what role can nurses play in this? You will need to think about the practical steps that are being (and can be) taken if this is the direction the NHS should go in.

Conclusion

Healthcare research needs to establish further whether teamworking actually occurs in any real sense and improves patient experiences as it is seen as *the* way to go for organisations. Teamworking is thought to bring many benefits to the workplace both in terms of efficiency and effectiveness as well as improving the working experience of staff. The challenge for nursing, with its own history, culture and knowledge base, is to see its place as an equal part of the wider healthcare team. More importantly for you is how you see your place in the team and how you experience becoming a team player. You will be assessed in practice on your ability to contribute to and be an active part of a team. To do this, not only do you need to develop knowledge around the human sciences (biology, physiology and anatomy, for example), and not only will you learn practical clinical skills, but also you need to know how you and others act, behave and think. You have to become socially skilled and develop a personal psychology that supports your journey through a complicated maze of interpersonal relationships. The next chapter will address some of the ideas and ways of thinking that we all adopt in our attempt to make sense of other people.

C H A P T E R   S U M M A R Y

This chapter introduced the idea of 'teamwork'. This has become a key idea drawn from the business, management and commercial worlds, and is applied to the NHS. This explores the difference between groups and teams, how teams function and the application of this to nursing work. You will need to decide to what extent nurses work in teams and whether any of this matters. An important idea is to think about whether the patient experience is enhanced by the way professionals work together. This chapter also introduced ideas that may be useful when you begin to address nursing leadership and management at the clinical level, i.e. in practice settings.

Activities: brief outline answers

Activity 5.1: Critical thinking (page 107)

Whether two parallel hierarchies exist in clinical teams in 2008 (13 years after the study) can only be observed and experienced by practitioners and/or updated research. However, evidence from other studies suggests that this may not be a far-fetched notion to apply still.

Is hierarchy a bad thing? This depends on a number of factors that apply. For example, a strict team hierarchy in an emergency situation may actually save lives as roles should be clearly understood and undertaken quickly without debate.

The third question is intended for students to reflect on.

Activity 5.2: Reflection (page 108)

You will need to identify the differing groups you belong to as a student nurse but look at the staff you work with and begin to identify any team characteristics. A good start is identifying if there is any group purpose. This may be easy at first; staff may talk about 'patient care' as the primary focus, but dig a little deeper, listen to what people say, watch what they do, look for contradictions or supporting actions. Think also beyond glib statements like 'patient care'. What exactly does that mean?

Activity 5.12: Critical thinking (pages 128–30)

There is not a right answer to this but maybe the phrase 'We are human beings. Ignore the interior workings, the strivings and desires, and team failure is inevitable' is a big clue. The NHS is a big organisation with many demands made upon it. The staff who make it run are human beings first and foremost, each with hopes, emotions and desires. We all bring frailties and strengths. Subsuming this humanity into the needs of a larger machine may miss the importance of recognising who we are and what we are about. This could be about our philosophical stance towards the world of work, i.e. is nursing a humanistic endeavour and/or is it about getting the work done regardless? You decide.

Activity 5.13: Critical thinking (page 131)

- One way is to identify how mistakes are dealt with. Is there a blame culture or do we look for a system as well as individual errors? So, does the team hold meetings to reflect on issues in practice as a way of learning?
- The clinical manager (ward sister/charge nurse or equivalent) is often seen as a key role in this regard. Mentors of practice are increasingly important as well.
- Learning? Well, this is a 'biggy'. A start is to divide it up into three: knowledge (cognitive), skills (psychomotor) and values/emotions (affective).

Knowledge review

Now that you've worked through the chapter, how would you rate your knowledge of the following topics?

	Good	Adequate	Poor
1. Teamwork.			
2. Belbin's team roles.			
3. Tuckman's team stages.			
4. Domains of learning.			
5. Effective healthcare teams.			
6. The learning organisation.			

Where you are not confident in your knowledge of a topic, what will you do next?

Further reading

Banks, C (2002) Making the most of your team. *Nursing Standard*, 17(10): 96.

Belbin, RM (1981) *Management Teams: Why they succeed or fail.* Oxford: Butterworth.

Belbin, RM (2003) *The Belbin Team Role Model.* Available online at www.belbin.com.

Tuckman, B and Jensen, M (1977) Stages of small group development. *Group and Organisational Studies* 2: 419–27. Available online at www.gmu.edu/student/csl/5stages.html.

Useful websites

www.businessballs.com Businessballs is a free ethical learning and development resource for people and organisations, run by Alan Chapman in the UK.

www.infed.org/leadership/leadership.htm Different models of leadership and the theory and practice of developing learning in organisations.

www.institute.nhs.uk NHS Institute for Innovation and Improvement (NHSII).

www.nwlink.com/~donclark/index.html Big Dog and Little Dog's Bowl of Biscuits – Don Clark's site in the United States.

Chapter 6

Understanding people, understanding yourself

Draft NMC Standards for Pre-registration Nursing Education

This chapter will address the following draft competencies:

Domain: Communication and interpersonal skills

2. All nurses must use a range of communication skills and technologies to support person-centred care and enhance the quality and safety of healthcare. They must make sure that people receive all the information they need about their care in a language and manner that is right for them, and that allows them to make informed choices and consent to treatment.
4. All nurses must take account of verbal and non-verbal communication and understand how these can be affected by factors such as disability, ill health, culture, age, ethnicity, gender, religious beliefs and socio-economic status. They should then respond in a helpful way towards people, their carers and their families.

Domain: Nursing practice and decision making

2. All nurses must listen, recognise and respond to an individual's physical, social and psychological needs. They must then plan, deliver and evaluate technically safe, competent, person-centred care that addresses all their daily activities, in partnership with people and their carers, families and other professionals.
5. All nurses must recognise and interpret signs of normal and changing health, distress or capability and act promptly to maintain or improve the health and safety of others.
7. All nurses must know when a person of any age is at risk and in a vulnerable situation in any environment and in need of extra support and protection. They must also act to safeguard them against abuse of any kind.

Draft Essential Skills Clusters

This chapter will address the following draft ESCs:

Cluster: Care, compassion and communication

4. People can trust a newly qualified graduate nurse to engage with them and their family or carers within their cultural environments in an acceptant and anti-discriminatory manner free from harassment and exploitation.

Draft Essential Skills Clusters continued

By entry to the register:

v.   Is acceptant of differing cultural traditions, beliefs, UK legal frameworks and professional ethics when planning care with people and their families and carers.

5.   People can trust the newly registered, graduate nurse to engage with them in a warm, sensitive and compassionate way.

By first progression point:

ii.   Takes into account people's physical and emotional responses when engaging with them.
iii. Interacts with the person in a manner that is interpreted as warm, sensitive, kind and compassionate, making appropriate use of touch.
v.   Evaluates ways in which own interactions affect relationships to ensure that they do not impact inappropriately on others.

By entry to the register:

vi.   Anticipates how people might feel in a given situation and responds with kindness and empathy to provide physical and emotional comfort.
viii. Listens to, watches for, and responds to verbal and non-verbal cues.
x.   Has insight into own values and how these may impact on interactions with others.
xi.   Recognises circumstances that trigger personal negative responses and takes action to prevent this compromising care.

Chapter aims

After reading this chapter you will be able to:

- understand how we begin to perceive others;
- uncover a few causes of misunderstanding and prejudices;
- understand how we present ourselves to others;
- explore the idea of emotional intelligence.

Introduction

Previous chapters have focused on the bigger picture; on those factors that are largely out of your control. We have looked at such things as the policy 'drivers' for inter-professional working; the context of the NHS; working with patients and clients; the relationship between professional groups; interprofessional learning; and what being in a team may mean and what an effective team could be. Finally, we need to look at ourselves to understand how we think to create our own values, beliefs, skills and attitudes in order to work with others more effectively. We have learned that effective collaboration involves the structure, the process and the culture of healthcare. The cultural element involves the internal thought processes we use in everyday experience as well as the social influences. If we can begin to understand how our minds work and how we go about forming impressions of others, we may begin to reflect on our actions in a more self-critical manner when we start making judgements about other people.

You will note that NHS structures and processes at your stage of experience may be difficult to change. However, during your first year as a student nurse you will be working on your personal and professional development. This means improving your communication skills, knowing the professional, ethical and legal constraints to clinical practice and developing sound working relationships. It will also mean developing skills of 'reflective practice'. As this topic will be covered in your curriculum, we will not address it here, except to say that it is argued to be a way of getting at and applying 'tacit' knowledge, i.e. knowledge that is in the background of your mind.

Therefore, we will now address the 'ways of thinking' (cognitive processes) that we all use and your personal development and the mental (thinking and emotional) tools you need. What follows is *not* an exhaustive discussion of the various insights and methods for developing this understanding. It is an introduction to various methods of getting to grips with how we are with each other, where our misunderstandings come from, and what we may try to do to change potential unhelpful behaviours and attitudes. The disciplines of sociology and psychology deal with many more theories than it is possible to discuss in this chapter. You will no doubt be exploring some of those theories in much more detail as part of your education. The aim within this text is to point out how these theories can help you in your work with other professionals and on your own.

Social perception

As soon as you meet people you will begin the often unconscious process of perceiving them in particular ways. You need to make almost immediate sense of the situation, the other person and the social context in which you find yourself. You will come into this encounter with an array of preconceptions, beliefs, values, etc. This may feel like an immediate experience. However, it is suggested (Fiske, 2004) that we have psychological and social filters that we use to process the information we receive. We attempt to explain, predict and control to some degree or other the social encounter. The filters we use will guide our control of this 'encounter' with others. We then *select* certain information and clues, *organise* these into understandable wholes and then make *inferences* about people based on this process.

Activity 6.1   *Reflection*

Remember when you first met the other students in your year group. What clues were you looking for? What ideas did you have to pick up about those students that you may become friends with? Having met the group for a while, have you begun to categorise other students according to, for example, their proposed branch of nursing? Did you focus on and select certain characteristics and traits? Did you put some of this information together to build a picture of the person in front of you? Can you remember making any inferences about who they are according to this picture you had built up?

While the process may have started when you first met, it is obvious that this process goes on as you continue to make selections, organisations and inferences.

Now think of a patient you have recently met. Did you go through similar thinking and perceiving? Describe a first encounter with a patient. Make comments about what you first thought.

As the results will be based on your own observation and experience, there is no outline answer at the end of the chapter.

Scenario 6.1

Selection: Upon meeting 'Phil' in his home following a referral from his GP, the Community Psychiatric Nurse (CPN) has already been given a selection of information, which would include things like age (43 years), any previous medical history (many previous in-patient admissions following self-harm), any previous contact with health and social services (the list is very long), or any current prescribed medications (anti-depressants). Walking into the house, the CPN will be bombarded with information that may give clues to Phil's current lifestyle (lives alone), mental health and social problems. Some things are discarded as useless information, while others are attended to. Phil's room may have many unwashed coffee cups and dirty plates, old newspapers on the floor, full and overflowing ashtrays, leftover cartons from several takeaway meals, etc.

Organisation: To make any sense of this, the CPN needs to organise this information from his or her observations – the cups, plates, newspapers, ashtrays, etc. This information may be organised into the category of 'unkempt house'. The CPN may have also selected information about Phil himself – unshaven, dirty fingernails, lank hair, body odour, etc., which may be organised into 'personal neglect'.

Inferences: From this process of selection and organisation, the CPN may start to make inferences – e.g. due to the 'unkempt house' and 'poor personal hygiene' – that Phil's mental health has deteriorated to the extent that his ability to care for himself has become difficult.

From this over-simplified example you will note that what happens in actual practice is far more complicated, especially if the CPN is going to make *correct* inferences.

It is helpful to try to understand how we perceive ourselves and others as this process will impact on the way we act towards others. Gross and Kinnison (2007) suggest the following key points as a means of understanding this process.

- We may be classified into four broad categories of thinker in relation to others: consistency seeker, naive scientist, cognitive miser and motivated tactician.
- Our overall impression of others is largely governed by *central traits* rather than *peripheral traits*.
- With strangers we use the *primacy effect*; with those we know well we use the *recency effect*.
- The *halo effect* is used when we have limited information about someone.
- We may have *implicit personality theories* (IPTs).
- *Stereotypes* – affect expectations – maybe create false illogical over-generalisations and influence behaviour.
- We actively manage the impression others have of us through impression management techniques/self-presentation. These include behaviour matching, appreciating/flattery, consistency in beliefs and matching verbal and non-verbal cues.
- We may be *high self-monitors* (matching behaviour to the situation) or *low self-monitors* (being yourself).
- *Self-disclosure* is affected by such things as reciprocity, norms, trust quality of a relationship and trust.

It may be fruitful to examine these ideas in more detail.

'We are all psychologists': ourselves as 'thinkers'

We are all psychologists. In attempting to understand other people and ourselves, we are informal scientists who construct our own intuitive theories of human behaviour. In doing so, we face the same basic tasks as the formal scientists.
(Nisbett and Ross, 1980)

How we view the social world and engage in behaviour with others is influenced in some ways by our memory, what information we pay attention to, what information we discount, change or ignore, and how others (individuals, groups, society and culture) affect our thinking and behaviour. How we do this has been outlined as a series of *metaphors* that describe the 'human being as thinker'.

The consistency seeker

People need to resolve inconsistencies in thoughts and behaviours. We have already noted the theory of cognitive dissonance (CD), which highlights that we seek consistency in our social and mental worlds. This suggested that people could not have thoughts or behaviours that are inconsistent with one another. For example, people cannot simultaneously believe that drug taking is bad but continue to smoke cannabis. CD theory suggests that inconsistencies between thought and behaviour are disturbing and motivates the person to resolve the inconsistency. This is done either by changing the behaviour ('I'll stop smoking 'spliffs') or changing the thought ('cannabis is not that harmful anyway').

Consistency applies to relationships with other people. For example, if your partner is not liked by a long-time friend whom you value, there is an inconsistency in the relationship. You need to restore this imbalance by adjusting your relationship in some way with the other two people. Stockwell's (1972) description of the 'unpopular patient' may also throw up inconsistencies – the difference between what your colleagues say about the patient and your own experience after spending time with them.

You will come across many of these differences with clinical colleagues and patients as you get to know people. You will then adjust your thinking and behaviour in an attempt to resolve them.

The naive scientist

This person likes to gather data about other people around them to arrive at a logical decision. This mimics the sort of method that a scientist may use to test hypotheses. The gathering and analysis of social information is a search for the cause of behaviour and it assumes a rational method of data analysis. In your education you will be introduced to ways of understanding people from a scientific approach and you may carry some of this understanding into everyday life. Many current discussions of criminal behaviour (whether it be knife use among young men in cities or prostitution) by lay people, which includes many healthcare staff, will centre around understanding such things as social deprivation or exclusion. An encounter with an alcoholic may involve analysis for clues as to the cause of the current problematic health behaviour based on such theories.

As a student you will begin to try to understand human behaviour from a lay/naive scientist perspective. As you learn more about the various explanations for behaviour, you may start to apply more thought-out explanations. For example, note what you currently understand about 'addictive' behaviour – how much of that knowledge is based on scientific theory and practice?

The cognitive miser

This metaphor sees people as being limited in their ability to gather, organise and process the information about the social world. In previous chapters we came across heuristic thinking in clinical decision making, i.e. the use of 'short cuts'. For example, if we wish to learn if a particular GP is approachable, knowledgeable and helpful, we can read their CV, observe them, ask their colleagues about them, watch them work with patients and obtain written references, visit other GP surgeries for comparison or discover their particular speciality. However, we will mostly not have the time, inclination or capacity to gather or organise this information. Hence the use of a short cut: we might ask a family member for their experience and opinion or we may simply 'like the look' of the person! When choosing a restaurant in a strange town we can make an internet search and read reviews. However, we can take a short cut by looking at the number of cars in the car park and asking ourselves 'is the restaurant busy?'

Your judgement about a well-groomed young child admitted for a common childhood illness, who nonetheless presents him- or herself as very reserved, may be based on assumptions about dress and demeanour that might actually obscure issues around child abuse in middle-class families. You do not have the time, experience or inclination to fully gather the information regarding potential non-accidental injuries. Your short-cut assessment leads you not even to consider the possibility.

Another short cut that we use to determine if a decision or choice or viewpoint is correct is to get consensus from others. This is based on the idea that consensus (i.e. 'if most people believe it') implies correctness (i.e. 'then it must be true'). Short cuts can result in both accurate judgements or biases and errors of judgement.

The motivated tactician

This assumes that we have multiple ways and methods available that enable us to make decisions about the social world and that we choose methods based on our goals, motives, or needs. For example, we may be motivated to maintain the positive regard of important people, colleagues and patients to whom we feel accountable. Our methods for interaction and decision making will change depending on who we are dealing with. We may be 'all things to all men'. Short cuts may be appropriate in some social situations. Part of your clinical practice assessment may focus on your ability to interact professionally and personally with others. If you have a limited repertoire – if you are socially inept or inexperienced – you may not be able play the motivated tactician. Your personal and professional development will depend partly on your ability to function at a high level in these social interaction skills.

Activity 6.2   *Reflection*

- At your next patient encounter, think to yourself about the methods you are using to understand both the patient and yourself in that role. Do any of the four metaphors apply? For example, on approach are you already making assumptions, looking for clues and short cuts? Are you a cognitive miser?
- Apply the four ways of thinking to Scenario 6.1 on page 138. How would any of the metaphors, if adopted by the CPN, affect the judgements made about Phil?

As the answers will be based on your own observation and experience, there is no outline answer at the end of the chapter.

The use of central traits

The suggestion is that we use particular information we possess about someone (*central traits*, which affect our evaluation of other traits) to gain an overall impression of who they are. Gross and Kinnison (2007, p144) refer to Asch's classic study of 1946 to illustrate this point. We may assess someone on the basis of certain central traits that impress upon us who we think they are. For example:

Person A is:	Person B is:
• Intelligent • Skilful • Industrious • Warm • Practical • Cautious	• Intelligent • Skilful • Industrious • Cold • Practical • Cautious
Rating	Rating ....

Rate persons A and B on a scale of 1 to 10, with 1 being negative and 10 being positive. Now rate A and B in terms of:

• generosity;
• sociability;
• wisdom;
• happiness;
• reliability;
• good-naturedness;
• politeness.

In Asch's experiment one group was given person A to rate, while a second group was given person B. Note that A is the same as B except for the description 'warm'/'cold'. Both groups were given a second list of 18 adjectives (such as those above) and asked to underline those that they thought applied to their person. The result was that two groups consistently chose different words according to their original rating of the person. The warm (A) person was seen as generous, sociable, etc. Those who only had B's traits (cold) used different (opposite) traits. Polite and blunt were substituted for warm/cold, with almost identical results. The conclusion is that warm/cold is a central trait that we use to judge someone as likeable, friendly, kind, etc. In a similar study, Kelley (1950) told one class that a lecturer was cold and another class that the same lecturer was warm. Both classes saw the same lecturer giving the same lecture. Those who expected a warm lecturer were more likely to engage in discussion.

Why should we do this? According to Asch, warm/cold impressions affect the other traits, but not all traits act in this way. Warm/cold are central traits and thus have this effect.

Is 'caring' a central trait? Nurses are supposed to be 'caring'. Do you think patients still hold on to this trait in their understanding of the nurse? What does this mean for their interpretation of the nurse? Do you think caring is a central trait that affects how others see you? If not, what may be the defining traits for nursing?

Gender/sexuality/attractiveness

The central trait model may seem a simplistic model of human behaviour, and it is probable that the process is not that straightforward. We bring to any encounter our own values and motivations that will impact on the process of impression formation. We need to consider other factors, e.g. gender and sexuality. Chapter 4 discussed the doctor–nurse relationship highlighting how issues of gender may impact on the way professions form impressions of each other. Gender and sexuality may therefore play an important role in working relationships. It may not be politically correct behaviour but physical attractiveness (as a factor in gender relationships) may have an impact over and above the obvious.

Concept summary: Attractiveness

Devendra and Randall (2007) argue that *attractiveness conveys reliable information about a woman's age, health and fertility*, particularly the waist to hip ratio (WHR) as an indicator of this attractiveness. They suggest that there is evidence from the literature that attractiveness is an important determinant of inter-personal (as well as romantic) relationships (Langlois et al., 2000). To evaluate the WHR, they showed pre- and post-operative photographs of women who had undergone micro-graft surgery (taking fat from the waist and implanting it in the buttocks). Following this surgery the photographs were rated for attractiveness. They conclude that WHR is a key indicator of attractiveness.

The implication, therefore, is that female staff (and patients?) with the appropriate WHR may be seen as more attractive and that this attractiveness confers certain advantages.

However, Fisak et al. (2007) suggest that personality as well as appearance is a determinant in perceptions of attractiveness of body shapes. Study participants were given a range of personality information (either no information, or negative or positive information) and asked to rate different body sizes. One finding was that a wider range of body shape (female) was chosen as being attractive when positive personality information was given.

These findings suggest that we use a wide range of information to make judgements about people. The relative weight of each factor (attractiveness, personality) used by people is difficult to judge.

It could be suggested that, when a person is seen as attractive or unattractive, certain assumptions are brought into play. In many cultures what is considered beautiful is also assumed to be 'good'. Alongside this, attractiveness may be associated with extroversion, and attractive people assumed to be possibly more popular and happy and possess attractive personalities (Dion et al., 1972). However, this could be due to a self-fulfilling prophecy. From a young age, attractive people may receive more attention, praise and encouragement; this then builds them up with a strong sense of confidence and self-worth, leading to higher achievement (Cash et al., 1976; Clark and Mills, 1979).

Darbyshire (1986) cites several studies (Corter et al., 1972; Kelly and May, 1982; Bordieri et al., 1983, 1984; Richardson et al., 1985) that support the hypothesis that 'beauty = good' in healthcare settings. Among the factors that affect how patients are treated by nurses is 'appearance'. It was also suggested that physically attractive children were held less responsible than less attractive children for disturbances, the behaviour being blamed on emotional causes. It may not be a one-way street, of course – the extra attention and praise may predispose the attractive to narcissism and vanity.

Lorenz (2005) reported on a survey of 11,000 people and suggested there was a difference in relation to their earnings between groups who described themselves as either attractive or less attractive. Those who described themselves as physically attractive earned more than the other group. People in the group who described themselves as less attractive earned, on average, 13 per cent less. Another factor was being overweight, the penalty for which was around 5 per cent. It is important to note that other factors such as self-confidence may explain or influence these findings as they are based on self-reported attractiveness as opposed to any sort of objective criteria. However, as a person's self-confidence and self-esteem are largely learned from how they are regarded by peers while growing up, even these considerations would suggest a significant role for physical appearance.

The discrimination or prejudice towards others based on their appearance is referred to as 'lookism' (Tietje and Cresap, 2005).

CASE STUDY: IS LOOKISM UNJUST?

LOOKISM is prejudice towards people because of their appearance. It has been receiving increasing attention, and it is becoming an important equal-opportunity issue. People we find attractive are given preferential treatment and people we find unattractive are denied opportunities. According to recent labor-market research, attractiveness receives a premium and unattractiveness receives a penalty. For both men and women, results 'suggest a 7–9-percent penalty for being in the lowest 9 percent of looks among all workers, and a 5-percent premium for being in the top 33 percent' (Hamermesh and Biddle 1994, p. 1186). Similar results were found in a study involving attorneys (Biddle and Hamermesh 1998, pp. 172–201).

(Tietje and Cresap, 2005)

So far, we may understand that our perception of the other person may have something to do with a trait we are told they possess or a trait we think they may possess. In addition, their gender/attractiveness may also influence our behaviour towards them and our understanding of their abilities.

Another factor to take into account is the *order* of things, also known as the *primacy–recency effect*.

- **Primacy effect**: 'first impressions count' – the greater impact of what we learn first about someone.
- **Recency effect**: the impact of what we learn later on.

Being told about a patient's irritability or impatience first at a handover before getting any other details may colour your perception of that patient. Gross and Kinnison (2007) argue that a negative first impression may be more difficult to alter than a positive one. They suggest that this may be due to a negative impression carrying more weight as it carries undesirable traits. It may be more adaptive (better) for us to focus on negatives because they are potentially more harmful or threatening to us.

Luchins (1957) suggested that the primacy effect may be stronger for people we first meet. The recency effect comes into play with people we know well. This may explain why we may retain first impressions of patients because in many cases we do not see them for long or the care episode is bound by time and the carrying out of a task. Those patients we really get to know allow the recency effect to alter our first impressions.

Activity 6.3   *Reflection*

- Identify an occasion when you altered your impression of someone when more information later came to light. How often have you judged someone on the basis of first knowledge?
- When you first enter a new clinical environment, consider whether primacy effects are being used to judge who you are. If so, how can you turn this to your advantage?

As the answers will be based on your own observation and experience, there is no outline answer at the end of the chapter.

The halo effect

In Asch's study the use of 'warm' in a list that produced more positive effects is an example of the *halo effect*. Simply put, if we are told someone is 'warm', we may then attribute other positive characteristics to them. The reverse is, of course, true for the description 'cold'. The halo effect is the idea that overall judgements about a person (e.g. 'she is likeable') affect the judgements about his or her characteristics or traits (e.g. 'she is intelligent'). Excellent examples of the halo effect are Hollywood film stars who, because they are usually attractive and likeable, are assumed to be intelligent, friendly and displaying good judgement. Reflect for a moment on who gets involved in global issues of poverty and global warming. Celebrities are often given platforms (as well as *take* platforms!) to pronounce on issues for which they may have no better training or education than you or I. Yet we listen – that is, until we come across (sometimes plentiful) evidence to the contrary that they may not be as intelligent or as well informed as we might otherwise have thought.

We may think that we could pick up these mistaken judgements by simple self-analysis and following our thought processes back to the original mistake. In the 1970s, a social psychologist, Richard Nisbett, set out to demonstrate how little access we actually have to our thought processes in general and to the halo effect in particular.

CASE STUDY: THE HALO EFFECT – THE LIKEABILITY OF LECTURERS

Nisbett and Wilson (1977) wanted to examine the way student participants made judgements about a lecturer. Students were told the research was investigating teacher evaluations. Specifically, they were told, the experimenters were interested in whether judgements varied depending on the amount of exposure students had to a particular lecturer. This was a total lie.

In fact, the students had been divided into two groups who were going to watch two different videos of the same lecturer, who happened to have

---

a strong Belgian accent. One group watched the lecturer answer a series of questions in an extremely warm and friendly manner. The second group saw exactly the same person answer exactly the same questions in a cold and distant manner. Experimenters made sure it was obvious which of the lecturer's alter-egos was more likeable. In one he appeared to like teaching and students and in the other he came across as a much more authoritarian figure who didn't like teaching at all.

After each group of students watched the videos they were asked to rate the lecturer on physical appearance, mannerisms and even his accent (mannerisms were kept the same across both videos). Consistent with the halo effect, students who saw the 'warm' incarnation of the lecturer rated him more attractive, his mannerisms more likeable and even his accent as more appealing. This was unsurprising as it backed up previous work on the halo effect.

Unconscious judgements

The surprise is that students had no clue whatsoever why they gave one lecturer higher ratings, even after they were given every chance. After the study it was suggested to them that how much they liked the lecturer might have affected their evaluations. Despite this, most said that how much they liked the lecturer from what he said had not affected their evaluation of his individual characteristics at all.

For those who had seen the cold distant lecturer the results were even worse – students got it the wrong way around. Some thought their ratings of his individual characteristics had actually affected their global evaluation of his likeability.

Even after this, the experimenters were not satisfied. They interviewed students again to ask them whether it was possible their global evaluation of the lecturer had affected their ratings of the lecturer's attributes. Still, the students told them it hadn't. They were convinced they had made their judgement about the lecturer's physical appearance, mannerisms and accent without considering how likeable he was.

(Jeremy Dean on PsyBlog, www.spring.org.uk/)

The halo effect is well used, and known, in marketing (Marconi, 2001) and the business world. Dean (2008a) states:

The halo effect in itself is fascinating and now well-known in the business world, books that have 'Harvard Classics' written on the front can demand twice the price of the exact same book without the Harvard endorsement. The same is true in the fashion industry. The addition of a well-known fashion designer's name to a simple pair of jeans can inflate their price tremendously.

Jeremy Clarkson of the BBC television programme *Top Gear* often points to the badge on a prestigious car to make the point that what is really sought after by car purchasers is the cachet of a car such as a BMW or Mercedes that the badge represents.

Whether the car is actually better on a range of objective criteria is often not the point.

Badges and symbols are short cuts to aid judgement about the worth of something or someone. What badges or symbols do healthcare professionals use to promote their own worth in the eyes of others?

Implicit personality theories

Gross and Kinnison (2007) argue that we all have our own theories about people – who they are, how we relate, how we should behave. They refer to implicit personality theories (IPTs). The trait theory is an example of an IPT, i.e. the use of traits by us is implicit in our judgements about other people. Physical appearance and attractiveness are also aspects of our personal theories. In addition, they discuss the importance of names and the use of stereotypes. An aspect of these IPTs is that they may be used as a way of quickly categorising or organising the information we are given about people.

Categorisation is about putting seemingly different things (and people) into groups or 'classes' in order to make sense of an otherwise senseless world. However, when we have done so, we then relate to those things or people according to the 'class' (ethnic group, economic class, age, height, weight, gender, sexual orientation, profession, diagnosis?) we have put them into, rather than relate to their individual characteristics. So, for example, two people who we perceive to be 'patients', or we consider to be of a certain age, are categorised according to this label even though we know of their individuality and uniqueness. The reason we downplay the individuality and relate more to the category is that to do otherwise would be overwhelming. If we respond to and focus on the uniqueness of everyone, we would be swamped by information.

In life, we need simple ways of identifying both objects and people. Categories help us to do this even when the category is misleading (Griffiths, 2000). Allport (1954) argued that categorisation *forms large classes and clusters for guiding daily adjustments* (p20).

As we grow and develop, we create in our heads 'pre-formed categories' to guide our daily perceptions and actions. These help us to make sense and guide expectations in social encounters. For example, when you attend a lecture you expect the teacher to behave in a certain way because you have a pre-formed idea of the category 'teacher' and thus you know what the norms of behaviour are.

Griffiths (2000) argues that, although categorising leads to simplification, it can also lead to *idleness and ignorance*. This relates to the 'cognitive miser' way of thinking. If we can slot someone into a category that we understand and are familiar with, we can bring our prejudgements into play and lessen the complication of trying to see the uniqueness of the person. Allport (1954) gives an example:

> If I can lump thirteen million of my fellow citizens under a simple formula: 'negroes are stupid, dirty and inferior' I simplify my life enormously. I simply avoid them one and all.
>
> (p21)

Therefore, we can see how categorisation can lead to prejudice based on stereotypes. Categorisation can be evidence-based using scientific principles, and as such may be open to criticisms and challenge. However, if it is based on hearsay, insufficient information, myth, legend and emotion, the scope for prejudice is rife.

Concept summary

Prejudice:

an opinion that is not based on reason or actual experience.

(COED, 2005)

a prejudgmental statement of ill doing, or an evaluation or decision made before the facts of a case could be properly determined and weighed . . . any unreasonable attitude that is unusually resistant to rational influence. Interpersonal hostility that is directed against individuals based on their membership in a minority group.

(www.bigot.eu/prejudice_en.html)

Stereotype:

a widely held but oversimplified idea of the typical characteristics of a person or thing.

(COED, 2005)

Social stereotypes:

a subcategory has a socially recognized status as standing for the category as a whole, usually for the purpose of making quick guesses about people and their qualities. For instance, the housewife-mother sub-category, though unnamed, exists. It defines cultural expectations about what a mother is supposed to be. In some cultures housewife-mothers are taken as better examples of mothers than nonhousewife-mothers.

(www.bigot.eu/social_stereotype_en.html)

- *Prejudices are abstract-general preconceptions or abstract-general attitudes towards any type of situation object or person.*

- *Stereotypes are generalizations of existing characteristics. These reduce complexity.*

(www.bigot.eu/prejudice_en.html)

Another aspect of categorisation is that it may be immune to contrary evidence. The prejudice that flows from this can be quite negative and hard to change. In the current debate about immigration into the UK, how much of it is based on actual knowledge of the people or the circumstances, and how much is based on emotion and fear? Think about drugs and drug use, and the category of 'addict'. How much is actually known by those who pronounce on drug policy (i.e. most of us), and how much of the evidence do we access, use or understand? In both cases, even if the evidence is clear and available, how many people will still adhere to their prejudices? We have had in recent history examples of whole nations falling under the sway of prejudice, categorising a certain ethnic group as *the enemy and destroyer of the purity of blood, the conscious destroyer of our race* and the exploiter of the worker as *the incarnation of capitalism, of the misuse of the nation's goods* (Joseph Goebbels).

CASE STUDY: NAMES AND STEREOTYPES

Stereotypical attitudes towards Christian names and gender may influence diagnosis

Wayne more likely to be viewed as malingering, feigning or personality disordered than Matthew

This study (Birmingham, 2000) aimed to investigate the effect of positive and negative stereotypical attitudes towards Christian male and female names on psychiatric diagnosis given to a young adult with psychiatric symptoms in police custody. The names were selected from the 150 most popular names in England and Wales (1974). Ten of the names were rated for attractiveness by psychiatrists blind to the study.

In a postal survey 464 psychiatrists were asked to give a diagnostic opinion on a young person with mental health problems in police custody. Four versions of the story were given and were different only by the name given to the person. Negative stereotype names were Wayne and Tracey, positive stereotypes were Matthew and Fiona.

Matthew received a diagnosis of schizophrenia significantly more frequently than Wayne (77 as opposed to 57 per cent). Wayne was more likely to receive a pejorative diagnosis (personality disorder, substance abuse, feigning, malingering) than Matthew (37 as opposed to 19 per cent). No significant difference was observed between the diagnoses given to Tracey and Fiona. Personality disorder diagnoses were more frequent with Fiona and Tracey compared to Matthew and Wayne.

Activity 6.4   *Reflection*

- If you have had children, reflect on the process of name giving. Did the names conjure up certain ideas, images or aspirations?
- To what degree does a name put someone into a category?

As the answers will be based on your own thoughts and experience, there is no outline answer at the end of the chapter.

Stereotyping is a form of categorising that is necessary to reduce the complexity of social life. The word itself may have a negative association as it commonly means a process that is illogical, false and harmful. However, if we need to categorise all things and people, the use of a stereotype may be a short cut to doing so. Allport (1954) accepted that many stereotypes may have some truth value to them. Stereotypes may simply be 'categories of people' and may actually serve an important purpose. Our social world is complex and difficult to understand. We do not have the time, experience or ability to deal with the wealth of information coming at us. Therefore we have to simplify the social world in order to deal with this information. Stereotypes are therefore *resource-saving devices* (Gross and Kinnison, 2007, p151).

- Are healthcare staff immune to prejudice and stereotyping? Are there categories of patient that lead staff to assume particular characteristics about an individual simply because they fit into a category (e.g. the category of 'drug user/substance abuser')?
- Do some diagnostic labels act as categories that define individuals so labelled?
- What is the difference between 'being a diabetic' and 'having diabetes?

An outline answer is given at the end of the chapter.

Stereotyping has been of interest in nursing (Evans, 2002; Muldoon, 2003; Andrews, 2004; Berry, 2004; de Carlo, 2007) and there are recent studies describing its effects. Ferns and Chojnacka (2005) argue from the findings in their study:

Media sexual stereotyping of the nursing profession is a well recognized phenomenon; however the sexual stereotyping of the image of the nurse by the sex/pornography industry is a much less publicized or discussed phenomenon within the nursing profession. Both national & local newspapers in the UK frequently use derogatory terminology to depict the sexual stereotyping of nurses. The media was found to emphasize both positive & negative nursing stereotypes and in comparison with other occupations & professions sexual stereotyping was prevalent.

(p1028)

Oxtoby (2003) argued:

there are many stereotypes within nursing, and while these can sometimes appear to be harmless banter or gentle interspecialty rivalry, they can also cause real problems for the profession.

(p34)

The suggestion here is that there are stereotypes _within_ nursing – ideas held by nursing specialities about other specialities, for example between critical care nursing, mental health and elderly care nursing.

Bradley and Jinks (2004) investigated the attitudes of two groups of newly recruited student nurses to gender and nursing stereotypes. The 1992 sample (n = 100) was a group of student nurses who were in their second day of studies of a Project 2000 type curriculum. The 2002 sample (n = 96) were in their second month of studies of a 'Fitness for Practice' curriculum. They used a questionnaire for measurement of attitudes to statements around gender and nursing stereotypes. They argued that there were significant differences between the characteristics of the two groups of students. The 2002 sample, it is suggested, had less of a propensity for beliefs in gender and nursing stereotypes than the 1992 sample. This was true of most statements related to gender stereotypes – i.e. nursing as 'feminine', male nurse stereotyping and issues related to nurses' uniforms.

De Carlo (2007) undertook an analysis of 19 American films produced between 1942 and 2005 to examine the portrayal of psychiatric nursing and psychiatric care in the cinema. The different images of male and female mental health nurses, power and authority and stereotypes of psychiatric patients are discussed. They conclude that Hollywood portrays the idea that mental health nursing _occupies an aberrant, secret and dangerous world and that its role remains that of custodial companionship_ (p338).

Stanley (1998) examines another stereotype of the male mental health worker as an abuser of female mental health patients!

Research summary

Levy et al. (2000) examined whether stereotypes of ageing might contribute to decisions the elderly make about when to die. Old and young participants (n = 64) were subliminally primed with either negative or positive stereotypes of old age and then responded to hypothetical medical situations involving potentially fatal illnesses. Consistent with their prediction, the aged participants primed with negative stereotypes tended to refuse life-prolonging interventions, whereas the old participants primed with positive age stereotypes tended to accept the interventions. This priming effect did not emerge among the young participants for whom the stereotypes were less relevant.

The results suggest that socially transmitted negative stereotypes of ageing can weaken elderly people's will to live. They also illustrate the level of influence that stereotypes can have on attitudes.

Impression management

It could be argued that, as soon as you meet someone else in your daily life, you begin to 'manipulate' the image of yourself that you are trying to put across to the other person. Sometimes this process is unconscious, but often it is not. There are rules, of course – conventions for social interaction that you learn as you grow up into an adult.

Goffman's (1959) *The Presentation of Self in Everyday Life* is a seminal work giving a detailed analysis of this process of 'mundane' social interaction. Goffman explores the details of individual identity formation, group relationships and the impact of the social environment. For Goffman, social interaction is viewed as a 'performance', constructed to provide other people with impressions that we want them to have of us. This performance exists regardless of our consciousness. How we establish our own social identity begins with the idea of a 'front' – a standard characteristic face we put to the world in order that others can characterise and interpret who we are. The front acts to allow others to understand us based on projected character traits.

Goffman calls this *dramatic realization* through the activities of *impression management*. In putting forward a front, information about us is given off through a variety of communication methods, all of which must be controlled to effectively convince others of the appropriateness of our behaviour.

Activity 6.6   *Reflection*

- Identify two different social settings, e.g. at home with your family and starting a new clinical placement.
- What methods do you use to ensure other people get the impression of you that you think is appropriate?
- Think about the language that you use, for example.

An outline answer is given at the end of the chapter.

So, how do we go about this impression management; how do we build our 'fronts'? We must be able to see ourselves as others see us to manage this impression. It is the ability to step into others' shoes that allows us to negotiate this process. Gross and Kinnison (2005, p155) outlined communication methods involved in impression management.

1. **Behaviour matching** is the attempt to attend to and copy the other person's behaviour. Formality by someone else may be matched by your own formality.
2. **Conforming to situational norms** means that we need to know what the appropriate behaviour is for the given social setting, in order to adopt the group's norms. One quick way to experience this is to break the norms. Try calling a consultant 'mate', for example!
3. **Ingratiation** in the form of flattery or appreciating others may elicit a favourable response. However, beware of sycophancy.
4. **Consistency** in beliefs and attitudes may be seen as favourable and increase your likelihood of a positive impression. Quickly changing behaviour or opinions will lead to negative impressions.
5. **Matching your own verbal and non-verbal behaviours** means that, if what you say does not match how you look, your true feelings may be given away. The non-verbal clue is often then taken as the true message. Try making a positive comment about your friend's expensive new outfit while at the same time grimacing. Which message will be received?
6. **Self-promotion** of your talents and abilities may be seen as a desire to be competent, but can be interpreted as pushy, arrogant and conceited.
7. **Intimidation** implies 'don't mess with me', but empty threats lose credibility.
8. **Exemplification** is the need to be seen as worthy, moral and saintly. Overdone, it is seen as being sanctimonious or 'holier than thou'.
9. **Supplication** is the method of last resort, and the aim is to be seen as helpless (strategic incompetence). The downside is a perception of being lazy, calculating and manipulative.

Working with your mentor

As a student nurse your experience with others will be guided, of course, by the social environment in which you find yourself. One of your tasks will be to complete a favourable practice assessment. Again, this is more than just learning certain practical tasks and clinical skills. It is about how you relate. You will be actively engaged in impressing upon others a positive image, and you and your mentor will be working on this aspect of your practice. If you have the skills of reflection and the ability to see yourself as others see you, this will assist with this activity. A useful tool to help begin this process is the Johari window.

The Johari window

'Johari' refers to Joseph Luft and Harry Ingham, who developed a communication tool to assist individuals and teams to begin the process of building trust through self-disclosure. It is aimed at improving understanding between people in a team or group setting. It is based on three principles:

- disclosure;
- self-disclosure;
- feedback.

This assumes that individuals can better understand each other by improving trust by disclosing information about themselves and learning about themselves through feedback from others.

The individual is represented by a box diagram of four quadrants (see Diagrams A and B):

1. **The open area**: this is the 'you' that you are aware of and others know also.
2. **The blind area**: this is the 'you' that others see and know but you do not.
3. **The hidden area**: the 'you' that you hide from others.
4. **The unknown area**: things that you and others are not aware of.

The way to build trust and open communication with others is to tell and ask. Self-disclose and get feedback so that the boundaries of the open area go down and across.

Diagram A: This represents someone new to a team, someone with poorly developed social skills, someone overly shy or someone who does not trust others. If you don't tell or ask, the open area remains small.

Open area	Blind area
This area is known both to yourself and to others. Don't tell, don't ask	Unknown by you but known by others.
Hidden area Known to you but not to others	**Unknown area** Unknown by both you and others.

Diagram B: This represents an established member of a team; someone willing to engage in the 'soft skills' of working with others. The aim is to try to make the open area as large as possible. You and others will journey along a path of shared discovery if you both ask and tell, if you self-disclose and seek feedback. You will experience self-discovery by asking others about yourself.

Open area	Blind area
This area is known both to yourself and to others. Tell others about yourself – self-disclose. Ask others about yourself – get feedback.	Unknown by you but known by others.
Hidden area Known to you but not to others	**Unknown area** Unknown by both you and others.

When developing a learning contract with your mentor, you will have specific learning outcomes to meet. However, part of this process will be to interpret often broad statements in a particular clinical setting. For example, you may be assessed against your ability to 'communicate effectively' with patients. Johari may be useful to think about because, if you have a large unknown area concerning your ability to communicate, neither you nor your mentor will be able to make accurate plans and assessments about your true abilities.

To really begin to understand your personal skills and knowledge about communicating with patients and co-workers, you both have to be prepared to engage in disclosure and feedback to increase the open area. This can be threatening as well as empowering.

Use the quadrants to base questions about your ability to communicate. For example:

- **The hidden area**: What is it you know about yourself that your mentor does not, that will impact on your ability to communicate? Are you naturally shy and reticent about discussing bereavement?
- **The blind area**: By definition there is something about your communication that you do not know. Perhaps you are over-familiar with patients in an attempt to cope? Or do you use inappropriate language picked up in other care settings (use of pet names for the elderly) that you thought is 'normal'?

In this way, agree that you are both trying to increase the open area and decrease the unknown. You are both engaged in an agreed process of feedback and disclosure. It is not about negative criticism but about growing as a person and as a professional.

James Manktelow (2003) makes the following suggestions:

Don't be rash in your self-disclosure. Disclosing harmless items builds trust. However, disclosing information which could damage people's respect for you can put you in a position of weakness.

Be careful in the way you give feedback. Some cultures have a very open and accepting approach to feedback. Others don't. You can cause incredible offence if you offer personal feedback to someone who's not used to it. Be sensitive, and start gradually.

(www.mindtools.com/CommSkll/JohariWindow.htm)

Self-disclosure partly determines how accurate a picture others see of you. It is the voluntary process whereby you offer information that others would not otherwise be able to access. This is done by both acts of commission (what we say and do) and acts of omission (what we *don't* say and do). Self-disclosure is not just about deep and meaningful issues in a bid to become closer, more intimate in a trusting relationship. It is also about sharing information about the everyday instances and likes that bring people together. This is just as important in building social ties. This is a skill that has to be learned and reflected upon.

Too much disclosure too early is off-putting. When introducing yourself to your new mentor in practice, you will not share detailed information about your last birthday party, your collection of stick insects or the colour of your underwear.

We are disclosing because we are managing the perceptions others have of us; we may want them to like us. Collins and Miller (1994) suggest that:

- people like those who share intimate secrets more than those who are secretive;
- if you like someone, you will disclose;
- you are more likely to like someone with whom you have shared secrets.

There will be times when your patients are in need of disclosure; at other times they will want to keep within themselves. A key skill of the nurse will be knowing the difference.

When others are disclosing, the way you respond will impact hugely on whether this develops or dies. Dean (2008b) suggests that people want to be 'understood' not just 'heard' and thus how your responsiveness, timing and attentiveness are crucial in helping this process along. You may want to think about how nurses interact with patients along these lines. In what situations can this ability to encourage disclosure on behalf of patients flourish? What helps and hinders this? For example, is there a gender difference? Are women more able/skilled at disclosure than men?

Self-monitoring

How much do you attend to the way you act, speak and behave on social situations? How much do you try to understand the norms of behaviour? To what degree do you refer to the social setting as a guide as opposed to your own internal mental state?

Snyder (1974) developed a self-monitoring scale based on a series of questions to which one responds 'true' or 'false'. For example, a high self-monitor would answer 'true' to the following statements.

- I guess I put on a show to impress or entertain people.
- When I am uncertain how to act in a social situation, I look to the behaviour of others for cues.
- I would probably make a good actor.
- In different situations and with different people, I often act like very different persons.

The following statements would elicit a 'false' response from a high self-monitor.

- I find it hard to imitate the behaviour of other people.
- My behaviour is usually an expression of my true inner feelings, attitudes and beliefs.
- At parties and social gatherings, I do not attempt to do or say things that others will like.
- I can only argue for ideas that I already believe.

High self-monitors concern themselves with behaviour that is socially acceptable. They will look for cues as to how to behave, attending to the speech, manner and the dress of others as a guide. Therefore, they may well behave differently in the various situations in which they find themselves. Hyacinth Bucket (pronounced 'Bouquet') would be a high self-monitor.

Low self-monitors remain themselves regardless of the social setting, and rarely adopt the norms of behaviour of that setting. Their own needs and values are their guides. Homer Simpson would be a low self-monitor.

Clinical practice demands both conformity *and* challenge. The high self-monitor in you may readily conform to what the normal group practice is; the low self-monitor in you may be more willing to challenge group practice. Both states have their place; the skill lies in knowing when it is appropriate.

Activity 6.7	Group work

With a small group of fellow students (4 or 6 in total is ideal), discuss the following questions.

- When is it appropriate to be 'oneself' in clinical practice?
- What patient interactions call for being genuine about who you really think you are, and when is playing a role more important?

- In breaking bad news to a patient (about their prognosis, treatment or diagnosis), to what degree do you need to be 'genuine', using your own self as part of the therapeutic relationship you are building?

As the answers will be based on the outcomes of your discussion, there is no outline answer at the end of the chapter.

Attribution

In understanding how we form impressions of others and judge causes of behaviour, we all engage in attribution. We do this intuitively, making judgements about them as a person and setting them in a situation. We make judgements about the causes of behaviour, locating those (internal) causes as something to do with the 'person', while locating the (external) causes in the setting in which the person finds him- or herself. We attribute the causes of behaviour in this way to make sense of the encounter. Nurses do this all the time with both patients and their colleagues.

Consider the angry, uncooperative, aggressive patient. Is this behaviour due to internal causes, i.e. the personal characteristics of the person that lead them to be this way with people, or external causes, i.e. because they find themselves in a strange environment, out of control and in pain?

According to Gross and Kinnison (2007, p159), there are six different traditions that form attribution theory:

- Heider's (1958) common-sense psychology;
- Jones and Davis's (1965) correspondent inference theory;
- Kelley's (1967, 1972, 1983) covariation and configuration models;
- Shachter's (1964) cognitive labelling theory;
- Bem's (1967, 1972) self-perception theory;
- Weimer's (1986) attributional theory of motivation.

The literature is extensive on this understanding of perception and impression formation. See Gross and Kinnison (2007, Chapter 9) for a full discussion. It is beyond the scope of this book to explore all these theories fully. You will not at this stage of your education need to be able to quote 'chapter and verse' of this literature. It is enough to be aware of the body of work that has been done on this subject and to address some of the ideas, for example *fundamental attribution error* (FAE).

We engage in FAE when we overestimate the internal and personal factors, and downplay situation factors when attributing causes of behaviour. We 'see' the person, but we 'don't see' the situation. It may be most noticeable that we are doing this when we attribute a behaviour to a single cause in the person themselves. An extreme example can be found in the case of Dr Harold Shipman, who murdered elderly people because he was, as a person, 'evil'. The patient mentioned above could be labelled as 'aggressive'. This is an aspect of who this person is and it is this aggressive personal characteristic that is the cause of their behaviour. On the other hand, it might be the situation that has caused the aggression. The environment may be anxiety provoking, which is then manifested in a display of anger/aggression.

The aggressive behaviour is the *foreground visible* aspect, while the *background* is less visible. We may easily judge this person on what we see. We did not see, however, a less than attentive receptionist, a patronising doctor, a long waiting time, fear about the possible consequences of the particular illness, treatment phobias, poor hospital experiences in the past, hunger, thirst, cold, pain, etc.

When the patient encounter is brief, there may be the tendency to need and use short cuts to understand the patient. FAE may result because we do not or cannot attend to the background features of behaviour. In other settings where we can get to know the background we may have more opportunity to learn about and attend to the background. This applies equally to colleagues as it does to patients.

There are ways of reducing this bias.

- Think about and attend to the 'consensus' of behaviour. If other people behave in the same way in similar situations, it may be that the situation is more likely to be the cause.
- Ask yourself, 'how would I behave in that situation?'
- Look for unseen causes; specifically, look for the background factors.

Cognitive biases

FAE is one form of 'cognitive bias', i.e. it is a way of thinking that leads to misunderstandings about other people. The following are some other examples of cognitive biases.

- **Self-serving bias**: This is the tendency to underemphasise the influence of your situation and overemphasise the influence of yourself. You pass an examination because of the study you have put in, the knowledge that you have and the level of understanding you have acquired. The opposite situation is that you fail because the teaching was poor, the assessment was not explained or the computer crashed. Success is down to you, but failure is down to someone else.
- **Dunning-Kruger effect**: There is incompetence in the methods used to become successful at activities. This incompetence leads not just to failure but to misunderstanding *the reasons* for that failure. The incompetence works in these two ways and does not allow understanding of the real reasons for failure. It leads to false thinking that 'all is well', or 'it is someone else's fault'.

    So, the inability to analyse a research paper accurately leads to not realising that an inaccurate understanding is created. A study is then critiqued on false grounds. For example, a small-scale qualitative research study (e.g. ten patients interviewed about their experiences of a diagnosis of cancer) is criticised for not producing results that can be generalised to the wider population. The writer making this statement does not realise that this sort of study cannot and does not set out to generalise from only ten patients. He or she will effectively criticise a lemon for not being a pear, but will not realise it. That is the first incompetence. If this judgement was based on poor study techniques or an inability to understand research ideas and this inability is not realised, i.e. the student thinks he or she can understand the ideas quite well, then this is the second incompetence. The student will blame failure not on his or her own inabilities but on, for example, poor teaching.

    A senior believes a junior colleague is incompetent because he or she does not quickly come up with the answers to particular questions about patient care. The real reason for the junior staff member's behaviour is incompetence by the senior in the methods of asking for the answers to questions (for example, by being brusque, aggressive, intimidating and not realising it). The senior's inability to see his or her own incompetence in asking patient care questions will prevent him or her from seeing where the true error lies.

Other cognitive biases include:

- **egocentric bias**: this may occur when someone claims more responsibility for the results of a joint action than an objective observer would;
- **herd instinct**: a tendency to adopt the opinions, and follow the behaviours, of the majority to feel safer and to avoid conflict;
- **illusion of transparency**: overestimation of your ability to know other people and their ability to know you;
- **in-group bias**: membership of a group may result in preferential treatment – 'us and them';
- **just-world phenomenon**: the world is 'just' and therefore people get what they deserve;
- **projection bias**: to assume unconsciously that others share the same or similar thoughts, beliefs, values, or positions;
- **self-fulfilling prophecy**: the tendency to engage in behaviours that elicit results that will (consciously or not) confirm our beliefs.

This list is not exhaustive, but what it illustrates is that our thinking processes are open to many different forms of error and bias. In developing critical thought we need to be able to understand that our thinking may not be as rational and evidence-based as we think it is, and to begin to develop ways of thinking that personally challenge ourselves to clarify our errors. This is one reason why *reflective practice* is emphasised in nursing.

If you are interested in the ways people engage in reasoning and their use of poor argumentative techniques, see Julian Baggini's 'bad moves' on the butterflies and wheels website (www.butterfliesandwheels.com/badmoves.php).

Emotional intelligence

In Chapter 5 we briefly discussed the concept of *emotional intelligence* (EI), a term derived from the work of Goleman (1995). Alan Chapman (www.businessballs.com) takes this idea on and discusses the *emotional quotient* (EQ), which puts this idea alongside the *intelligence quotient* (IQ). The core idea of EQ could be understood as *awareness, control and management of one's own emotions, and those of other people*.

EQ has two components:

- understanding yourself, your goals, intentions, responses and behaviour;
- understanding others, and their feelings.

Goleman (1995) identified the five 'domains' of EI as:

1. knowing your emotions;
2. managing your own emotions;
3. motivating yourself;
4. recognising and understanding other people's emotions;
5. managing relationships, i.e. managing the emotions of others.

By working on these domains and developing them within yourself and others, you may become more productive and successful in your endeavours. Other outcomes from this focus are:

- stress reduction;
- conflict resolution and management;
- improving working relationships.

Emotional work may involve a degree of acting at a surface or deep level (Hochschild, 2003). The surface actor knows that the smile, the caring attitude, the touch are professional acts, undertaken to achieve a particular end, e.g. patient comfort and well-being. The deep actor undertakes these things as part of who they are – the skills and attitudes come naturally or have been developed to such an extent that they just *are*. Deep acting involves deceiving yourself (you are not aware of the 'act' if indeed it can still be called an act) as well as others in order to carry out the emotional work, while surface acting deceives only others.

From this perspective, the nurse's personal development as a human being is as important as the acquisition of technical skills. Empathy and the 'therapeutic use of self' are tools in the nurse's skill box that assist with exercising and developing emotional intelligence. Learning about how human beings interact, about our own values and needs in working life is therefore core, not peripheral, to nursing practice.

This cuts to the essence of many nursing models and philosophy, in that the nurse should not be an automaton working on an assembly line as if dealing with inanimate objects. Nursing, as a discipline, discusses and claims to be based on individualised humanistic care that is person-focused (Roper et al., 1980), holistic (Roy, 1980), interpersonal relationship building and a therapeutic use of self (Peplau, 1988), caring as part of moral consciousness and the collective responsibility to support and care (Orem, 1985) and claims to have ethical, personal, aesthetic as well as empirical dimensions (Carper, 1978).

Much of nursing theory thus focused on the nature of interpersonal relationships as the key aspect of nursing work. Emotional work (Smith, 1992) can be seen as the link that binds this all together. If this is true, becoming emotionally intelligent would be a key skill. The corporate world of management may be adopting this model of thinking applied to developing more effective teams within organisations whose primary purpose is bottom line-driven, i.e. they have to satisfy their customers and their shareholders. Paradoxically, the idea of EQ comes from a discipline other than nursing.

Emotional work for nurses is challenging. It calls on personal resources that we may not wish to commit (or know we have) to what could be for many 'just a job'.

Conclusion

This chapter has only scratched the surface of the theories and the knowledge base that is available to help us understand ourselves and others. We have tried to discuss the thinking processes from the individual's point of view to show that everything is not quite as it seems. You will need to think about the interactions you will experience with people and move beyond simple explanations. You will need to be able to pick your way through an emotional minefield if you are going to protect yourself and your patients from undue stress and burn-out. In the future, you will be in positions of leadership. When you are, the behaviour you model will be examples for those following on. What you pass down will help to define what modern nursing will become. To help with this you will need to grasp fully the personal nature of working with others in organisations and you may wish, in the future, to further your studies by learning from several perspectives and theories such as the following.

- **Transactional analysis** This is a model for learning about emotional responses that apply in all areas of life (E Berne (1966) *Games People Play*. London: Deutsch).
- **Psychodynamic approaches to leadership and management** These approaches show an understanding of conscious and unconscious emotional 'drivers' that affect behaviour and attitudes (M Kets de Vries et al. (2007) *Coach and Couch: The psychology of making better leaders*. Basingstoke: Palgrave Macmillan).

- **Transformational leadership**: This is a model for leading that places value on individuals, supporting them in decision making and creative problem solution (BM Bass (1990) From transactional to transformational leadership: learning to share the vision. *Organizational Dynamics*, 18 (3): 19–31).
- **Corporate social responsibility**   This is the idea that organisations exist not only to fulfil core business objectives (be they increasing sales or meeting targets such as the reduction of waiting times), but that they have a wider responsibility to society and the individuals who work for them (*Corporate Social Responsibility: A government update*, available online at www.csr.gov.uk).
- **Empathy and personal growth**   Working life for individuals can only progress and be healthy if the personal elements of work are addressed and developed (see the seventh habit of S Covey (1989 and 2004) *Seven Habits of Highly Effective People*. London: Free Press).
- **Sustainability**   Whatever we do socially, politically or economically, can we leave enough for the future or are we wasteful? This includes addressing consumption patterns. Do we need to use the amount of the earth's resources that we currently do? (See *UK Sustainable Development: What is it and how can I do it?*, available online at www.sustainable-development.gov.uk/what/index.htm).

See also Alan Chapman's website (www.businessballs.com), where much of this material can be found condensed.

This list is by no means exhaustive but one thing the points have in common is the need to work closely with others to bring about the desired results.

Modern organisations address 'work–life balance' ideas, accepting that the most important asset they have is the staff who work for them. How much this is window dressing or an aspiration, rather than actual practice, is, of course, a matter for investigation at the 'coal face'.

Working with other people can be challenging, distressing, embarrassing, complex and downright nasty. It can, of course, be the opposite as well – life enhancing, joyous, satisfying and affirming. If you wish to nurse, you will embrace it all.

CHAPTER SUMMARY

This chapter introduced some of the sociopsychological processes we use as individuals in our everyday life in an attempt to uncover how we (sometimes unconsciously) relate to one another. This is about understanding yourself to realise how you make judgements about people and how this affects how you behave towards others. Whereas Chapter 4 suggested some social influences that affect behaviour and attitude, this chapter has taken a more individual perspective. The focus has been on such things as the 'implicit personality theories' that we use in our relationships. It is important to note here that nursing is as much about the use of 'soft skills' as it is about the achievement and mastery of technical competencies. An understanding of such things as emotional intelligence brings the art and science of nursing together.

Activities: brief outline answers

Activity 6.5: Critical thinking (page 149)

- 'Normal rubbish': The accident and emergency (A & E) department has for many years been used as a source of primary care. However, patients attending the A & E department with needs that could have been met by their GP have tended to be pejoratively labelled by staff as inappropriate attendees. Jeffrey (1979) reports the labelling of patients as good patients or 'normal rubbish', describing how nurses make value judgements about patients based on limited knowledge. The judgements are often in respect of the patients' social worth and the nurses' own perceived roles. He argues that A & E staff have a basic understanding of their role; therefore, when they are asked to treat patients seen as outside their role they view them as illegitimate. Is this view still valid?
- Being diabetic (asthmatic, epileptic) is a defining (almost permanent) label about who you are. It assumes your whole being and humanity is viewed through this lens. It can be a comforting label or it can be disabling, making you less than human. Having diabetes may assume that you are a human being first and foremost who just happens at this point in time to experience particular symptoms; it does not define your essential humanity.

Activity 6.6 Reflection (page 150)

Your first day in the clinical setting. You ensure that your clothes are clean and ironed. Your hair is in place and you have paid especial attention to personal hygiene. You start by not talking too much or being over-familiar; in fact, you listen more than usual to pick up on the social cues. Think what would impress you about a newcomer to the team, and mirror that behaviour. Of course, if you are not skilled in this everyday activity you could get this horribly wrong.

Knowledge review

Now that you've worked through the chapter, how would you rate your knowledge of the following topics?

	Good	Adequate	Poor
1. Social perception.			
2. Ourselves as thinkers and cognitive bias.			
3. Central traits and lookism.			
4. Gender, sexuality and attraction.			
5. Implicit personality theories, the halo effect, impression management and stereotyping.			
6. Emotional intelligence.			

Where you are not confident in your knowledge of a topic, what will you do next?

Further reading

Bordens, K and Horowittz, I (2001) *Social Psychology*. Mahwah, NJ: Lawrence Erlbaum Associates.

Gross, R and Kinnison, N (2007) *Psychology for Nurses*. London: Hodder Arnold.

Stewart, I and Joines, V (1987) *TA Today: A new introduction to transactional analysis*. Nottingham: Lifespace.

Useful websites

www.businessballs.com Businessballs is a free ethical learning and development resource for people and organisations, run by Alan Chapman in the UK.

www.infed.org/leadership Different models of leadership and the theory and practice of developing learning in organisations.

www.nwlink.com/~donclark/index.html Big Dog and Little Dog's Bowl of Biscuits – Don Clark's site in the United States.

Chapter 7

Interprofessional education for collaborative practice

Draft NMC Standards for Pre-registration Nursing Education

This chapter will address the following draft competencies:

Domain: Professional values

8. All nurses must be responsible and accountable for keeping their own knowledge and skills up-to-date through continuing professional development and life-long learning. They must use evaluation, supervision and appraisal to improve their performance and enhance the safety and quality of care and service delivery.

Domain: Communication and interpersonal skills

1. All nurses must communicate safely and effectively to forge partnerships and build therapeutic relationships with people, family members and groups. They must take individual differences, capabilities and needs into account, and respond in a non-discriminatory way.
5. All nurses must recognise and respond effectively, using therapeutic principles, to people who are anxious or in distress in order to promote wellbeing and manage personal safety. They must know when other specialist interventions may be needed, including independent advocacy services, and make the referral.

Draft Essential Skills Clusters

This chapter will address the following draft ESCs:

Cluster: Care, compassion and communication

1. As partners in the care process, people can trust a newly registered graduate nurse to provide collaborative care based on the highest standards, knowledge and competence.

By first progression point:

i. Articulates the underpinning values of the NMC *Code* (2008).
ii. Works within limitations of the role and recognises own level of competence.
v. Is able to engage with people and build caring professional relationships.

Draft Essential Skills Clusters continued

By entry to the register:

xiv. Uses professional support structures to develop self-awareness, challenge own prejudices and enable professional relationships, so that care is delivered without compromise.

7. People can trust the newly registered graduate nurse to protect and keep as confidential all information relating to them.

By entry to the register:

vii. Acts appropriately in sharing information to enable and enhance care (carers, MDT and across agency boundaries).

10. People can trust the newly registered graduate nurse to deliver nursing interventions and evaluate their effectiveness against the agreed assessment and care plan.

By entry to the register:

x. Reviews and makes adjustments to the care plan with the person and in response to evaluation, communicating these changes to colleagues.

11. People can trust the newly registered graduate nurse to safeguard children and adults from vulnerable situations and support and protect them from harm.

By first progression point:

ii. Shares information with colleagues and seeks advice from appropriate sources where there is a concern or uncertainty.

By entry to the register:

vi. Shares information safely with colleagues and across agency boundaries for the protection of individuals/the public.

Chapter aims

After reading this chapter you will be able to:

- understand the meaning, aims and potential benefits and challenges of interprofessional learning;
- reflect on opportunities for interprofessional learning in the practice setting.

Introduction

This chapter examines the ideas and evidence of the perceived value in being involved in shared and interprofessional education, and how it aims to make a difference on a number of levels for nurses and other health and social care professionals, relevant public sector services and ultimately for the care that patients receive. It includes consideration of the meaning of 'interprofessional education' in the context of the previously discussed and related concepts of professional values and attitudes, teamworking, organisational culture, skills and generic competencies, and the nature of collaboration and collaborative practice.

Activity 7.1   *Critical thinking*

What is your understanding of the term 'interprofessional education'?
Write down your own definition, and then look up the term in textbooks and on the internet. Write a paragraph summarising the information you have found. How does your definition compare to those you have found?

There is an outline answer at the end of the chapter.

The meaning of shared education

Shared education, sometimes described as multiprofessional education, is defined broadly in this chapter as the shared events and experiences of learning by students, or can be defined as *occasions when two or more professionals learn side by side for whatever reason* (Centre for the Advancement of Interprofessional Education (CAIPE), 1997). This is also frequently referred to as 'common educational experiences', meaning that in health and social care there is a broad base of generic knowledge, skills and attitudes that all professions and the wider public sector services share. While learning through a 'shared' approach does not imply that it is structured as interprofessional education, an opportunity for incidental learning about other learners of professions still exists.

Activity 7.2   *Reflection*

Take a moment to think about a time when you have experienced 'shared learning' with others who have similar or different interests; that is, when you joined with students or learners from other courses or disciplines as part of the preparation for entry into your nursing, in another and previous programme, or activity elsewhere.
One example might be that of joining with a group for information technology in your A level or Access course.

- What was the general topic of your learning?
- How was the class or group organised?
- What teaching method was used?
- Was there an opportunity to discuss any course-specific issues?

A brief outline answer is given at the end of the chapter.

The benefits of shared education

Shared education is sometimes set up and timetabled to accommodate large numbers of students who have the same generic learning needs. This means that the session is usually held in a lecture theatre or similar venue and delivered by a teacher or lecturer who is the subject specialist. These formal arrangements can be useful for receiving information. However, they could be a hindrance to individual or group interactions and therefore do not necessarily enable you to learn about others, except through incidental learning when questions are asked or examples invited from the lecturer.

Even so, where students come together to learn generic subject material and knowledge about health, social care and other related areas, there is still potential for learning from others through the social aspect of the experience. Try to visualise shared learning as the first step on the ladder, with interprofessional education as the second step and collaborative practice as the third step, as follows:

| 3. collaborative practice |
| 2. interprofessional learning |
| 1. shared (common/multidisciplinary) learning |

Having considered the meaning of shared education, let's move on to the idea of interprofessional education and consider how its structure and process can influence your learning.

A definition of interprofessional education

In contrast to shared or multidisciplinary education, defined as *occasions when two or more professionals learn side by side for whatever reason* (CAIPE, 1997), the definition widely accepted in the UK for interprofessional education (IPE), also provided by CAIPE, is: *when two or more professions learn with, from and about each other to improve collaboration and the quality of care* (CAIPE, 1997, 2002).

The World Health Organization (WHO, 2010) has adapted the well-established CAIPE definition to apparently show a slight perspectival and pragmatic change that affects the priorities of IPE, stating that *IPE occurs when students from two or more professions learn about, from and with each other to enable effective collaboration and improve health outcomes* (p9). You will note that the outcome of IPE is broader in this definition. It extends beyond the quality of care to improve health outcomes for people and populations.

IPE involves learners or students from different professions coming together to learn through the use of a range of appropriate resources (often scenario-based and competence-focused) about each other's professions and the way in which their respective roles contribute to effective and evidence-based patient care. For IPE to take place, it is necessary for there to be students with patients and peers or qualified professionals from more than one profession in the same setting, whether that be face to face or online through a discussion forum. It can be driven by learning outcomes and require students to actively engage in an educational experience, student-directed and managed or through a learning contract; or it can be highly structured, engaging students in a formal, documented and assessed experience.

Gilbert (2005) proposes that:

Notions about collaboration inform and drive interprofessional education and should lead to sustainable system changes within centres of advanced education that ensure a permanent place for interprofessional education in all health and health sciences programs.

Clemow and Parker (2006) suggest that a core set of principles or philosophy for IPE can underpin the learning experience so that learning is meaningful and authentic, and where students, other learners and patients/service users can benefit through the experience. When students are brought together to learn without clear aims and learning outcomes in IPE, it can lead to frustration and resentment that time is being taken out of their curriculum for something that is pointless and irrelevant to their profession.

Broadly, the aims of IPE (DH, 2000, 2006; CAIPE, 2005, 2007; WHO, 2007; Clemow and Parker, 2006; WHO 2010) are:

- to prepare and develop professionals who can work in an interprofessonal team in order to respond to local health need, and deliver safe and effective support, intervention and care;
- to enable effective collaboration and improve health outcomes;
- to contribute a generic curriculum for all professionals and staff;
- to redesign ways of working in order to address the new ways in which care is to be delivered;
- to mitigate the global health workforce crisis.

Derived from a systematic review undertaken by Barr et al. (2005), three components to IPE have been identified that are complementary, overlapping and correspond in part with each other in time, function and purpose. They are:

1. preparing individuals for collaborative practice;
2. learning for working in teams;
3. developing services to improve care.

A fourth category proposed by Barr (2007) was sourced from IP literature beyond those that met the original criteria for inclusion in their 2005 systematic review is: *improving life in communities* (p42). More research is required to test this proposition and provide evidence about whether this fourth element is a component of IPE and one that ultimately can have a transformative effect on society. In their systematic review of IPE outcome measures, Hammick et al. (2007) show that there is developing evidence for informing interprofessional policy making, education and practice, with an ultimate aim of transforming care and services. The WHO (2009) supports this proposition.

In summary, IPE ultimately aims to transform health and social care practice such that students and providers can learn, develop and deliver, so that patient/service users and carers can reap the benefit in improved health outcomes (WHO, 2010). Having identified these components or dimensions of IPE, we might assume that different activities will be required in order to produce the desired outcomes.

Activity 7.3   *Reflection*

Consider again the definition of IPE. Now reflect on your experience of IPE in your university or college programme.

- Who was present?
- Who perhaps was missing? What is your rationale for the answer?

Activity 7.3 continued

- Who else might have been there to make it a more meaningful educational experience?
- How did the lecturer organise the session and learning activity (e.g. small group discussions)?
- What made it an IPE experience as distinct from shared education? (See the earlier definitions.)

(Check your understanding against the WHO (2010) definition again – see page 165.)

- Did you learn with, from and about each other?
- What resources did you use for learning (patient scenarios or case histories, skills laboratory)?

As the answers will be based on your observations, there is no outline answer at the end of the chapter. Instead, a short commentary is given.

Likewise, you may have already experienced a practice placement as part of your professional programme and so could consider the questions above in that context also.

Having considered what shared education and IPE are as hierarchical categories (see page 108), we now move on to explore how these potentially impact on ways of working for achieving collaborative practice.

Collaborative practice

The concept of collaborative practice is based on the idea that excellent patient support, intervention and care rely on the expertise of several care providers and the patient/service user. Collaborative practice is considered to be a complex behaviour that *happens when multiple health workers from different professional backgrounds work together with patients, families, carers and communities to delivery the highest quality care* (WHO, 2009, p9). In previous chapters it has been shown that a number of factors affect the way individuals behave, react and communicate.

Some might argue that there is a quantum leap from IPE to collaborative practice. However, Martin-Rodriguez et al. (2005) propose that successful collaborative practice in healthcare teams can be attributed to a number of elements, including processes associated with interprofessional relationships in the team, the conditions within the organisation, and the organisation's environment. Furthermore, Zwarenstein and Bryant (2000), in their systematic review, reported that increasing collaboration promoted moderately improved processes of importance to patients. However, these require further research to confirm the findings and make any generalisations.

Because health and social care organisations rely on teamwork to provide effective support, intervention and care, it would seem most appropriate to focus IPE opportunities in the workplace team, such that it is authentic, contextualised and therefore meaningful. More research is required in this area so that a greater understanding can be gained of the processes and factors that affect the ability to transfer knowledge, skills and attributes necessary for collaborative practice.

Parcell et al. (1998) suggested that taking time to be involved in discussion and exchanges of views can enable learners to understand the roles people play in their health and social care work, and the way they think, feel and react as individuals and professionals. IPE aims to provide opportunities for this to happen through a range of learning and teaching methods. Methods that enable you to work collaboratively in teams with your peers, professionals and the public can be valuable in achieving this (WHO, 2009).

A significant proportion of nursing and other health professional learning time takes place in practice settings. Therefore, it is proposed that sociocultural and constructivist (see Jaramillo, 1996; Bleakley, 2006) learning theories and methods of learning that take into account the learning environment, including relationships between people, working in teams and the intelligent tools of practice, can be powerful in predicting and providing an explanation of how learning occurs in teams in health and social care contexts.

Concept summary

Socioculturalism and constructivism

- **Sociocultural approaches**: first developed by the Russian psychologist Lev Vygotsky in the first half of the twentieth century. They emphasise the interdependence of social and individual processes in the co-construction of knowledge.
- **Constructivist approach**: strongly influenced by Vygotsky's work, holds that people learn within a social context, through collaboration that enables greater understanding on the part of the individuals than would be possible through learning alone. So, to be effective, learning must include both social and practical elements.

In your practice placement, consider undertaking the following exercises to help you think about the opportunities for enhanced learning where professionals, agencies and the public work together. This can help you to develop an awareness of what is happening around you in the care setting and to reflect on it in terms of developing your competence in collaborative practice.

Activity 7.4   *Reflection and critical thinking*

In agreement with your mentor, shadow someone of your choice from a different profession or agency from your own. This means that you will take an opportunity to observe, ask questions and discuss support, intervention and care activities with another professional who you are not necessarily familiar with, and therefore gain an understanding of what their role entails in relation to the care of patients and as a member of the multidisciplinary team.

You might consider the following questions when undertaking this activity, reflecting upon it and in a subsequent discussion with your mentor.

- What are the role and responsibilities of the professional?
- What are the requirements for entry and qualification in his or her role?
- What is the professional's pattern or way of working?
- How does he or she contribute to the multidisciplinary team?

Activity 7.4 continued

- What activities did you observe the individual doing and how did he or she interact with the patient and/or carer?
- What surprised you about the role of the professional that you shadowed?
- Did your observation challenge your previous belief about the profession that the individual represented?

As you write a short reflective account for your portfolio, ask yourself: What happened there? What does it all mean? What do I do with that information? How has it affected me as a developing professional (nurse)?

As the results will be based on your observations and experiences, there is no outline answer at the end of the chapter.

Activity 7.5   *Communication and critical thinking*

Make a list of all the people who work in your practice placement area. Ask your mentor for some clues about who else works behind the scenes or in other departments (e.g. radiographer, GP, receptionist, porter, etc.).

Arrange with your mentor to attend a multidisciplinary team (MDT) meeting (a meeting where more than one profession is represented to discuss the care needs of a patient and/or carer), sometimes called a case conference. Observe and listen to communications, interactions and discussions between all those present.

Make notes on the following.

- Who was present at the meeting? Which professions did they represent and how many of them were there?
- Was the patient or carer present at the meeting?
- What was the content and purpose of the meeting?
- Who chaired and/or led the meeting?
- Who contributed verbally to the discussion?
- What non-verbal communication did you observe? Was it supportive of, or different from, the verbal communications?
- How were decisions made and who was involved in making them?
- Was there anything that seemed to be left unsaid?
- What was the general mood of the meeting?

Discuss your observations and the significance of what you observed in respect of the meaning of collaborative practice with your mentor. To capture what you learned from this activity you might want to write a reflective account and add it to your portfolio. To help with constructing this account, ask yourself: What happened there? What does it all mean? What do I do with that information? How has it affected me as a developing professional (nurse)?

As the results will be based on your observations and experiences, there are no outline answers at the end of the chapter, but we have made a brief comment.

Activity 7.6 — *Communication*

- Think about your own attitudes and behaviour in relation to other professionals and members of the care team.
- Observe and think about occasions when a professional refers a patient to another professional. Have you ever thought that this would not be possible if the one making the referral was unaware of what the role of the other professional was?
- There are four words, beginning with 'C', that are important in terms of IPE and working.
  - **Communicate**: What do you think it means for patients and for members of the health and social care team?
  - **Coordinate**: What does it mean to you? Who coordinates the care of patients in your practice placement?
  - **Cooperate**: What does it mean to you?
  - **Collaborate**: What does it mean to you?

Outline answers are at the end of the chapter. Your personal experience will further determine your responses.

Making interprofessional education work

Common occupational standards across children's practice linked to modular qualifications [will] allow workers to move between jobs more easily.

(DfES, 2004)

The way in which NHS staff work, and how they collaborate with each other in effective teams, is key to the delivery of patient services in the NHS.

(DH, 2005a)

A collaborative practice-ready health worker is one who has learned how to work in an interprofessional team and is competent to do so.

(WHO, 2010)

Calls for better teamwork and better liaison between professionals and agencies are not new. As far back as the 1980s, work was undertaken to try to establish the foundations of multidisciplinary working, yet no clear methods were evident as to how this might be achieved. However, current government and policy agendas are calling for a radical shift away from old-style teamworking to new ways of working on an interprofessional basis. This need for a change in the way professionals and health and social care agencies work together has led to the identification of IPE as a way of establishing and promoting collaborative practice. The debate continues about whether this is best delivered pre- or post-qualification, and how effective either of these would be in encouraging and supporting health and social care professionals and agencies to work together.

Effective IPE requires much more than students or practitioners from different professions simply listening together in shared lectures (Freeth et al., 2002). Participants need to work actively together on tasks for which they take joint responsibility in a natural environment. Therefore, arguably, IPE requires attention to team building among students (Gilbert et al., 2000) through effective communication, cooperation, coordination and collaboration, and among academics and practitioners/providers in practice areas. This requires a shift in culture in learning and teaching as well as in health and social care practices.

Multiple initiatives, policies and frameworks have subsequently been aimed at driving the IPE agenda forward to become mainstream, although it is recognised that professional bodies, colleges, societies and associations are somewhat behind in the shift. Examples of these initiatives include the establishment of the new regulatory bodies for the United Kingdom, that is, the Nursing and Midwifery Council (NMC), the Health Professions Council (HPC) and the General Social Care Council (GSCC); the reforms culminating in the NHS Knowledge and Skills Framework (KSF) (DH, 2004); and the establishment of the NHS Modernisation Agency (2004), which was designed to support flexibility in personal, career, role and service development, which have subsequently become the remit of the Skills Sector Council, Skills for Health/Care.

Further professional body developments and policy initiatives provide indicators of the commitment to learning for clinical effectiveness and making a contribution to the wider healthcare agenda through integrated professional and interprofessional education that develops knowledge, capability and competence (NMC, 2004a). The increased emphasis on streamlining processes for health and social care provides learning and teaching tools for IPE, such as process mapping, multidisciplinary and clinical care pathways, and the map of medicine.

A number of national IPE initiatives aimed to bring learners together to develop an appreciation of the generic elements of professional knowledge and practice. Some of these have been perceived, through experience, to be effective and reliable as well as challenging. The South West was one of the first of the NHS regions to report how it was implementing the partnership agreement between the NHS Executive and the Committee of Vice Chancellors and Principals (now Universities UK) that aimed to provide a shared commitment to the development and expansion of IPE, flexible pathways and joint career initiatives (Universities UK, 2003).

Most recently, with the overt commitment of the WHO to IPE through the new *Framework for Action on Interprofessional Education & Collaborative Practice* (WHO, 2009), a platform has been established for debate and action in developing and sustaining IPE in the mainstream and on a global basis, not only to serve the purpose of improving health outcomes through public involvement but also to address the global workforce crisis. One of the key messages in the framework is to propose that, after 50 years of research, the WHO and those associated with it believe that the examples and evidence are developing from many different countries, which leads to the conclusion that collaborative practice strengthens health service systems and improves health outcomes. They believe that these will be strengthened and supported by integrated health and education policies.

Activity 7.7   *Reflection*

Write down two reasons why you think it might be beneficial for different professionals (nurses, doctors, occupational therapists, dietitians, physiotherapists and others) to learn together. Then write down two reasons why you think it might be difficult to achieve.

Your answer will be based on your experience and reflection on learning throughout this chapter, so there is no outline answer at the end.

Barriers to effective IPE

The barriers to IPE are well documented and can be categorised on three levels, as reiterated by McPherson et al. (2001):

1. organisational matters, such as differences in academic policies and strategies between institutions and programmes, and financing;
2. the logistics of timetabling, resourcing and accessing, preparation of staff, student baseline entry variations, etc.;
3. people, relationships and attitudes, where competition rather than cooperation and collaboration exists, time and commitment to IPE, language and fear of dilution of professional identity, etc.

These barriers are seen to be heightened when the education programme is based in the university setting, and where a mix of students is timetabled to work together in placements where there is limited capacity to receive them and support them with, for example, adequate mentor support. Gilbert (2005) proposes that structural changes need to be made so that IPE, based on patient-centred collaborative practice, can be fully integrated into all health-related education programmes. IPE becomes essential when the patient/service user is engaged in decisions at the centre of professional focus, requiring care that is beyond the knowledge and skill of any one profession (NMC, 2008).

Overcoming the barriers

The creative use of social space, e-learning simulation and placement allocations can enable IPE. However, just because you are in the same placement, it should not be assumed that you will learn interprofessionally. The following example could be accessible through a real practice placement or through a virtual online, interactive world where you might assume the role of the patient, the nurse or any other member of the team and interact using skills of observation, negotiation and decision-making, among others.

Scenario 7.1

A community-based team, in which nurses work with other members, supports the care needs of a 67-year-old female patient with a long-term (chronic) health condition, such as chronic obstructive pulmonary disease (COPD). Due to the complex nature and associated health problems, a number of professionals and agencies will make up the team. As a student working alongside the Community Matron, for example, you might take the opportunity to discuss with the patient all the people and agencies involved in her care and get to know many of the professionals involved, how they work and the extent of their roles. They might include a community nurse, respiratory nurse, physiotherapist, social worker, care worker, pharmacist and others.

Observing and joining in a multidisciplinary case conference at the local health centre or in hospital will provide you with an experience that shows how they work together, and to what level the patient is included in the decision-making about her care. Or, having learned about COPD, you might visualise or

Scenario 7.1 continued

simulate the role of the patient, and 'experience' what it is like to live with the disease.

You are likely to see some good and not so good examples of professionals working and learning together for the purpose of improving the health outcomes of the patient.

A desired outcome might include reducing the risk of an exacerbation of the patient's condition and re-hospitalisation. In discussion, it might be shown how risk assessment, a self-care regime and availability of prophylactic medications and oxygen can help achieve this.

IPE is best achieved through *authentic processes* by which persons engage in learning to structure collective thinking towards collaborative health and/or social care (Clemow and Parker, 2006). This implies that IPE is grounded in authentic team-focused support and intervention, as collaborative practice, and emerges through patient empowerment and a collective mind (team). Through initial exposure to the concept of teamworking and systems, a number of interprofessional skills and conversations can be programmed and developed, drawing on specific criteria, care pathways and other health frameworks. This is supported by D'Eon (2004):

Learning in teams is best facilitated by the progressive mastery of more and more complex tasks incorporating the best practices of co-operative learning as part of the experiential learning process.

Concept summary: Authentic processes

Authentic means genuine, identifiable and recognisable.

The term as used here stems from the work of Taylor (1992), who presented his argument concerning his view of three malaises associated with our modern society:

1. loss of meaning;
2. disenchantment with the world, leading to instrumental reason (e.g. technology to solve problems even when other solutions seem more reasonable or possible, or risk assessment to determine financial savings);
3. the loss of freedom where, contrary to wider belief, choice is restricted due to political instrumentation.

Taylor's ideas are open to debate and can enable you to think about how people make sense of and develop meaning from their experience of illness, health and healthcare; the use of technology and pharmaco-genetics and their role in health; and people's access to health and the ability to make choices. As professionals, we have a responsibility to partner people and populations to improve health outcomes.

The principles of authentic IPE (Clemow and Parker, 2006) therefore might include:

- an inclusive environment that respects and values difference (people and professions);
- people at the centre of learning;
- engagement: care based on holistic care;
- preparation and support of people, materials and systems;
- authentic learning, teaching and assessment;
- a dialogic and constructivist approach to developing interprofessional identity and practice;
- development in practice, informing and informed by theory.

Several models of IPE exist and these are central to the debate about which stage of the curriculum is the most appropriate to implement these. For example, debate has occurred around the development of professional identities, or lack thereof, at the pre-registration stage, and what the role of IPE has in shaping identity. A study undertaken by Adams et al. (2006), which drew on a sample of 1,252 students in their first undergraduate year of health and social work where IPE was embedded in the programmes, showed that professional identity was evident before they started their programmes. This was attributed to a number of factors and variables, including gender, profession, previous employment or work experience in health and social care contexts, understanding of teamworking, knowledge of profession and cognitive flexibility. Furthermore, Horsburgh et al. (2006) describe how, in a study to determine the attitudes, values and beliefs towards clinical work organisation of students entering undergraduate medicine, nursing and pharmacy programmes in Auckland, findings indicated that, before students start their professional programmes, groups and subcultures differ in how they believe work should be organised. As a starting point for IPE this poses a number of challenges and potential barriers. Medical students believed that clinical work should be the responsibility of individuals, whereas nursing students have a collective view and believe that work should be systemised; pharmacy students were on a mid point in this continuum.

Different approaches

You might have experienced a number of approaches and methods in IPE; these are described in the literature as captured by Barr et al. (2005, 2006) and are useful to consider. These have been adapted to include:

- **exchange-based learning**, taking the form of group discussions, seminars and workshops in mixed groups;
- **action-based learning**, taking the form of action learning sets, problem-based learning and group problem-solving activities;
- **practice-based learning**, taking the form of learning in placements and through work experience;
- **simulation-based learning**, generally involving rehearsing relevant skills, role play and use of simulators, in a safe environment, e.g. skills laboratories;
- **observation-based learning**, entailing work shadowing or visits to relevant places to gain an understanding of how things work there;
- **e-based and blended learning**, usually occurring through online web-based activity, through video-conferences, virtual computer-mediated interdisciplinary teams or

'second life' activities that are usually carefully 'blended' with other teaching and learning methods;

- **clinical guidelines, policy and protocol development**, which involves examining current clinical practices by 'process mapping' to identify blocks and areas that can be improved in the patient journey through the care system. Analysis and work with integrated patient care pathways can also enable understanding of the need to work interprofessionally, since no one professional has the necessary knowledge to provide all aspects of care in all situations. The latter approach has become increasingly important in current health and social care practice.

There is a raft of opportunities for engaging with patients, carers, professionals and agencies to explore their contribution to health and social care in diverse practice settings. Referring back to an earlier exercise, you might reflect on the number of people who come into contact with just one patient during a short episode of illness in hospital or in the community. The patient is an 'expert' of their own experience, and all those professionals, other workers and carers provide an excellent context for IPL.

Students' experience of IPE

There has been a significant amount of evaluation of the effectiveness of IPE, much of which has been captured in Barr (2002). The majority of such evaluation has been from the student or educator perspective, with little if any examination of the impact or otherwise of IPE on the experience of patients. Key issues that have emerged from evaluations include the student's readiness for IPE, the timing of IPE, the content, delivery and assessment methods, and the lack of a theoretical framework. Furthermore, there is an ongoing debate about whether students need to become socialised into their chosen profession before they can usefully engage in IPE, or whether early involvement in IPE prevents the setting up of barriers that mitigate successful IP collaborative practice.

There has been little work on evaluating the effect of IPE on the care or service that is delivered from the perspective of the end user. A Cochrane systematic review failed to find methodologically sound studies to evaluate IPE and its effect on either professional practice or healthcare outcomes (Zwarenstein et al., 2000).

Barr (2002) commented on reviews of evaluative studies of IPL and concluded that the emerging evidence reiterated that IPE, in favourable circumstances and in different ways, can contribute to improving collaboration in practice. Traditional and expedient approaches to evaluation are valued. However, naturalistic methodologies will illuminate the human experience associated with IPL. The challenge is to undertake research and evaluation so that it informs IPE and development and, in particular, in practice settings so that it impacts on patient outcomes.

There is some evidence (Barr et al., 2005) that suggests there is an interlinked relationship in the three identifiable aspects of IPE: first, pertaining to individual preparation for collaborative practice whereby knowledge, skills and attitudes are developed through exposure to and engagement with other professions; second, the aspect of cultivating collaboration in organisations, communities and teams; and, third, the aspect that impacts on improving the service and the quality of care for patients. This includes implementing policy for flexibility and to improve quality of service and care, and as a result drive up recruitment and retention of staff. However, what is clear from the literature is that more research is necessary to provide more evidence of the impact of IPE and, in particular, its possible impact on patient outcomes.

New nurse preparation programmes and IPE

There are many challenges for undergraduate programmes in preparing graduates for redesigned healthcare practice, where the emphasis is on systemised work and team-based approaches. These include issues of professional socialisation, which begins before students enter programmes, selection of students, attitudinal shifts and IPE. IPE could become the mechanism for mutual learning through a social contract for the benefit of patients and as a means to enable transcultural competence, whereby diverse values, perceptions and ethnicity can be understood. The definition includes many different aspects within IPE, requiring a range of learning and teaching approaches and methods.

Attempts to classify IPE so that comparisons can be made between programmes and their outcomes is perhaps best seen in Barr et al.'s (2005) work, which involved an empirically grounded study from 107 robust evaluation studies included in a systematic review. As mentioned earlier in the chapter, they included three overlapping foci: preparing individuals for collaborative practice; learning to work in teams; and developing services to improve care. The evaluation studies were mainly those that were undertaken in North America, where the healthcare and education systems are considerably different from those in the UK; thus, the generalisability of the findings might be cautioned. However, they do provide a starting point for preparing an interprofessional curriculum. In 2007, Barr added a further focus/theme/aspect yet to be integrated into a wider conceptualisation of IPE, after drawing on sources in the interprofessional literature that did not meet the original review criteria. The fourth focus aspect that Barr offers is to improve the quality of life in communities and this will be discussed further.

Scenario 7.2

IPE in action

A female patient (Mrs Kaur) has a long-term health problem: type 2 diabetes with associated health issues (obesity, a venous leg ulcer and limited mobility). She lives alone, uses a mobility aid and is unable to get out of the house without assistance. She also needs help with personal care and hygiene.

The people involved in Mrs Kaur's care might include: Mrs Kaur herself, nurses (community matron/ community nurse/diabetes specialist nurse, practice nurse), general practitioner, home carer, podiatrist, pharmacist, social worker, Citizens Advice Bureau and housing personnel, and perhaps others. In authentic IPE for collaborative practice, you will learn about these multiple health and social professionals and workers from different backgrounds and experiences. This will enable you to develop knowledge about their roles and processes for working together with Mrs Kaur, her family, carers and agencies to deliver the highest quality care.

In an ideal situation, IPE through this scenario would take account of learning opportunities developed with the range of people involved in Mrs Kaur's care, either in the educational setting (seminar room, skills laboratory, through simulation with students of the different professions and agencies, and actors), through e-learning or in the practice setting. Shadowing and observing as well as questioning those involved will help develop your understanding of how they work as a team.

Conclusion

This chapter has considered the aims and outcomes of IPE with the potential for developing collaborative practice. It has provided the policy context that drives IPE and learning, and provides compelling evidence for sustaining and evaluating it so that there is clear evidence to know that it makes a difference in improving the quality of patient support, intervention and care. A shift is required away from IPE that is based on expensive unsustainable initiatives. Rather, IPE might best be achieved through the student taking control in seeking opportunities, using contextually created resources, and reflecting on their experiences, so that they can gain understanding of others' roles and how they might interact effectively within the multidisciplinary team for the benefit of patients, improving the services they require.

Activity 7.8　　　　　　　　　　　　　　　　　　　　　　　　　　　*Reflection*

Look back at Activity 7.6 and remind yourself of the four words beginning with 'C' that are important in terms of IPE and working:

- communicate;
- coordinate;
- cooperate;
- collaborate.

If you have experienced structured IPE as a learner, do you think it helped improve these four Cs? If you have not yet been involved in formal learning with other professionals, what do you think the experience might contribute to your understanding of these four Cs?

Do you think IPE is something you can experience, or even initiate, on an informal basis?

Your response will be based on your experience, developing understanding and reflection on your learning, so there is no outline answer at the end of the chapter.

Knowing that there are a number of barriers to IPE can enable responsive actions to mitigate against their impact and move towards a synergy between education and society. It is necessary for all health- and social care-related departments in higher education institutions to make education collaborative practice a priority and take measures to embed structures to support and sustain it. Principles of IPE have been described that can form the basis of an educational philosophy that empowers and places the patient at the centre of care and authentic learning experiences. More research is required to provide evidence on the relationship between IPE and collaborative working practice. The impact of the WHO *Framework for Action on Interprofessional Education & Practice* is yet to be realised; however, it goes a long way towards articulating best practice for shaping IPE. It provides educators, practitioners, agencies and policy makers with systems and processes for developing and sustaining IPE. It is believed to be the necessary step in preparing a *collaborative practice-ready health workforce that is better prepared to respond to local health needs* (WHO, 2010).

C H A P T E R   S U M M A R Y

This chapter examined the meaning and aims of interprofessional education (IPE) so that it is recognisable within your professional programme and makes its purpose understandable for the benefit of patient care. The differences between shared and interprofessional learning have been explored, leading to conclusions that, by reflecting on real-life practice experiences, the outcomes of interprofessional learning become more transparent and meaningful. This also serves to promote interprofessional learning opportunities because they become more readily identifiable.

The need for IPE has been set in the context of the National Health Service and World Health agendas and professional policies, with clear directives and initiatives to change the way in which health and social care and education are delivered – safely, effectively and flexibly – changing to meet the workforce need.

Over some time there has been a drive for increased autonomy in health and social care. IPE serves to promote autonomy and collective thinking and an understanding of roles and respect for service users, other professionals, and agencies. There are suggestions that creating an authentic environment for interprofessional learning is important, so that understanding and empowerment can be constructed. Consideration has been given to the application of principles for IPE, since they are more transformative than using models that are developed in and for specific contexts.

Activities: brief outline answers and reflections

Activity 7.1: Critical thinking (page 164)

In contrast to shared or multidisciplinary education, defined as: *occasions when two or more professions learn side by side for whatever reason* (CAIPE, 1997), the definition widely accepted in the UK for interprofessional education (IPE) is:

> *Inter-professional education occurs when two or more professions learn with, from and about each other to improve collaboration and the quality of care.*
>
> (CAIPE, 1997, 2002)

This means that interprofessional learning can take place in any setting where you can further develop knowledge and understanding about other professionals, agencies and yourself in relation to the needs of service users, their carers and their families.

Activity 7.2: Reflection (page 164)

As you reflect on the experience, you may know that you learned something from the other students, but probably didn't have the time or opportunity to discuss with them their specific course and topic in any depth in the class. This means that, while it was useful to be in the group to learn generic knowledge together (perhaps information technology), you may have come away from the session without any additional knowledge about how that subject was used in their discipline or course. If we look at it from this angle, it could be seen as a lost learning opportunity. However, by being in the same place with a larger number of other students, you will have invariably gleaned something from one or two people that you would not have, had you not been there at all. This means that you were involved in shared or common learning.

Activity 7.5: Communication and critical thinking (page 169)

This activity is based on your personal experiences, but you can find further reading references below. You can also discuss your experiences and findings further with another professional.

Activity 7.6: Communication (page 170)

- **Communicate**: defined as: to give or exchange information; to have a good personal understanding. Effective communication is a core competence and is at the heart of effective care. In all the damning reports mentioned earlier, there was a lack of communication that led to the failure of services to patients and clients.
- **Coordinate**: defined as: to organise a complex activity in which numerous people are involved and bring their contributions together to form a coherent or efficient whole. You can also refer back to Chapter 4 for more insights.
- **Cooperate**: defined as: to combine forces; to work or act together to achieve a common goal. If professionals cooperate with other members of the team there is a better opportunity for effective care because, as described at the outset of this chapter, all professionals have generic knowledge and skills that they share, so they can work across professional boundaries when necessary, thus creating a smooth pathway for the patient.
- **Collaborate**: defined as: to work with another person or group in order to achieve something. The WHO (2009) states that:

> Collaborative practice happens when multiple health workers from different professional backgrounds work together with patients, families, carers and communities to deliver the highest quality of care. It allows health workers to engage any individual whose skills can help achieve local health goals.

This, therefore, continues to recognise the need for staff to include patients and families. This comes in the context of a worldwide shortage of healthcare staff (Yan et al., 2007) and the need to introduce innovative ways of meeting global health needs. We know that any one profession does not have all the knowledge for safe and effective patient care. Therefore, at local, national or international levels, to collaborate with others in a team will mean collective thinking and shared decision making, and actions for effective care and service improvement. Furthermore, care pathways require that professionals work together and contribute expertise to the episode of care through the patient's journey.

Knowledge review

Now that you've worked through the chapter, how would you rate your knowledge of the following topics?

	Good	Adequate	Poor
1. The definition of interprofessional education.			
2. Why IPE is considered important.			
3. The outcomes you can expect from learning about, from and with other professionals, and working together with patients, families, carers and agencies.			
4. Opportunities for interprofessional education for collaborative practice during your programme.			

Where you are not confident in your knowledge of a topic, what will you do next?

Further reading

Centre for the Advancement of Interprofessional Education (CAIPE) (1997, updated 2002) *Interprofessional Education: A definition*. CAIPE bulletin no. 13. Available online at http://caipe.org.uk/index.php?&page=define&nav=1 (accessed 19 September 2006).

Centre for the Advancement of Interprofessional Education (CAIPE) (2006) *Effective Interprofessional Education*. Available online at http://caipe.org.uk/index.php?page=define&nav=1 (accessed 20 March 2008).

Finch, J (2000) Interprofessional education and teamworking: a view from the education providers. *British Medical Journal*, 321: 1138–40.

Quality Assurance Agency (QAA) (2006) *Statement of Common Purpose for Subject Benchmarks for Health and Social Care*. Gloucester: Quality Assurance Agency for Higher Education in England.

World Health Organization (WHO) (2009) *WHO Framework for Action on Interprofessional Education & Collaborative Practice*. Available online at www2.rgu.ac.uk/ipe/WHO_report_Interprofessional%20Ed%20Sep2509.pdf (accessed 8 January 2010).

Useful websites

http://caipe.org.uk The Centre for the Advancement of Interprofessional Education, this website includes a student section.

www.dh.gov.uk/en/Healthcare/Highqualitycareforall/index.htm Department of Health, with a link to High Quality Care for All.

www.nmc-uk.org The website of the Nnursing and Midwifery Council, with links to the review of pre-registration nursing calculation (2010).

References

Adams, K, Hean, S, Sturgis, P and Macleod Clark, J (2006) Investigating the factors influencing professional identity of first year health and social care students. *Learning in Health and Social Care*, 5(2): 55–68.

Adamson, B, Kenny, D and Wilson-Barnett, J (1995) The impact of perceived medical dominance on the workplace satisfaction of Australian and British nurses. *Journal of Advanced Nursing*, 21(1): 172–83.

Allen, D (1997) The nursing medical boundary: a negotiated order? *Sociology of Health and Illness*, 19: 498–520.

Allen, R (2004) These are a few of my favourite things: reflections on the doctor–doctor relationship. *Internal Medicine Journal* 35(1): 65–6.

Allport, G (1954) *The Nature of Prejudice*. Cambridge, MA: Addison Wesley.

Andrews, J (2004) Perceptions of nursing: confirmation, change and the student experience. *International Journal of Nursing Studies*, 41(7) (September): 721–33.

Aritzeta, A, Swailes, S and Senior, B (2007) Belbin's team role model: development, validity and applications for team building. *Journal of Management Studies*, 44(1): 96–118.

Asch, S (1946) Forming impressions of personality, in Gross, R and Kinnison, N (eds) (2007) *Psychology for Nurses and Allied Health Professionals*. London: Hodder Arnold, chapter 8.

Atwal, A and Caldwell, K (2005) Do all health and social care professionals interact equally? A study of interactions in multidisciplinary teams in the United Kingdom. *Scandinavian Journal of Caring Sciences*, 19 (September): 268.

Baggs, J, Schmitt, M, Mushlin, A, Mitchell, P., Eldredge, D, and Oakes, D, et al. (1999) Association between nurse-physician collaboration and patient outcomes in three intensive care units. *Critical Care Medicine*, 27(9): 1991–8.

Baird, J and Bradley, P (1979) Styles of management and communication: a comparative study of men and women, *Communication Monographs*, 46: 101–11, in Zelek, B and Phillips, S (2003) Gender and power: nurses and doctors in Canada. *International Journal for Equity in Health*, 2(1). Available online at www.equityhealthj.com/content/2/1/1.

Barr, H (2002) *Interprofessional Education: Today, yesterday and tomorrow: a review*. London: Higher Education Academy, Heath Sciences and Practice Network.

Barr, H (2007) Interprofessional education: the fourth focus. *Journal of Interprofessional Care*, 21(S2): 40–50.

Barr, H, Koppel, I, Reeves, S, Hammick, M and Freeth, D (2005) *Effective Interprofessional Education: Argument, assumption and evidence*. Oxford: Blackwell.

Barrett, G, Sellman, D and Thomas, J (2005) Interprofessional Working in Health and Social Care. Basingstoke: Palgrave Macmillan.

Batty, D (2003) Catalogue of cruelty. *The Guardian*, 27 January. Available online at www.societyguardian.co.uk.

Becker, H, Geer, B, Hughes, E and Strauss, A (1976) *Boys in White. Student culture in medical school*. Kansas City, KS: Transaction Publishers, University of Kansas.

Benner, P (1984) *From Novice to Expert: Excellence and power in clinical nursing practice*. Menlo Park, CA: Addison-Wesley.

Berry, L (2004) Is Image important? *Nursing Standard*, 23 (18 February): 14–16.

Beveridge, W (1942) *Social Insurance and Allied Services Report*. Presented to Parliament by command of His Majesty. London: HMSO.

Biggs, S (1997) Interprofessional collaboration: problems and prospects, in Day, J (ed.) (2006) *Interprofessional Working*, Expanding Nursing and Health Care series (ed. L. Wigens). Cheltenham: Nelson Thornes Cheltenham.

Birmingham, L (2000) Stereotypical attitudes towards Christian names and gender may influence diagnosis, in Gross, R and Kinnison, N (2007) *Psychology for Nurses and Allied Health Professionals*. London: Hodder Arnold. Also available online at www.rcpsych.ac.uk.

Bleakley, A (2006) Broadening conceptions of learning in medical education: the message from teamworking. *Medical Education*, 40(2): 150–57.

Bloom, B (1956) *Taxonomy of Educational Objectives: The classification of educational goals*. Susan Fauer Company.

Borch Jacobson, M (2005) A zero theory, in *Le livre noir de la psychanalyse*. Paris: Editions des Arènes. English translation available online at http://butterfliesand wheels.com (accessed 8 February 2008).

Boulos, MNK and Wheeler, S (2007The emerging web 2.0 social software: an enabling suite of sociable technologies in health and health care education. *Health Information and Libraries Journal*, 24(1): 2–23.

Bourbonnais, F and Baumann, A (1985) cited in Bucknall, T and Thomas, S (1997) Nurses' reflections on problems associated with decision making in critical care settings. *Journal of Advanced Nursing*, 25(2) (February): 229–37.

Bradley, E and Jinks, A (2004) Angel, handmaiden, battleaxe or whore? A study which examines changes in newly recruited student nurses' attitudes to gender and nursing stereotypes. *Nurse Education Today*, 24(2) (February): 121–7.

Brand, S (2006) Nurses' roles in discharge decision making in an adult high dependency unit. *Intensive and Critical Care Nursing*, 22(2): 106–14.

Brimblecombe, N (2005) The changing relationship between mental health nurses and psychiatrists in the United Kingdom. *Journal of Advanced Nursing*, 49(4): 344–53.

British Broadcasting Corporation (BBC) (2003) GP out of hours complaints soar. *BBC News*, 23 September. Available online at http://news.bbc.co.uk (accessed 8 February 2008).

British Broadcasting Corporation (BBC) (2006a) Half of NHS Trusts must improve. *BBC News*, 23 September. Available online at http://news.bbc.co.uk (accessed 8 February 2008).

British Broadcasting Corporation (BBC) (2006b) London: hospitals closure anger. Trench, Z, *The Politics Show*, 8 October 2006. Available online at http://news.bbc.co.uk (accessed 8 February 2008).

British Medical Association (BMA) (2005) Healthcare in a rural setting. BMA Board of Science, January 2005. Available online at www.bma.org (accessed 8 February 2008).

British Medical Association (BMA) (2008) Health professionals taking control on climate change. Available online at www.bma.org.uk/ap.nsf/Content/climatechange (accessed 25 March 2009).

Brown, G (2008) PM's New Year message to NHS staff. Department of Health, 1 January 2008. Available online at www.dh.gov.uk/en/DH_081585 (accessed 8 February 2008).

Bucknall, T and Thomas, S (1995) Clinical decision making in critical care. *Australian Journal of Advanced Nursing*, 13(2): 10–17.

Bucknall, T and Thomas, S (1997) Nurses' reflections on problems associated with decision making in critical care settings. *Journal of Advanced Nursing*, 25(2) (February): 229–37.

Camden, C. and Kennedy, C (1986) Manager communicative style and nurse morale. *Human Communication Research*, 12: 551–63.

Campbell, NC, Elliott, AM and Sharp, L (2000) Rural factors and survival from cancer: analysis of Scottish cancer registration. *British Journal of Cancer*, 82: 1863–6.

Campbell, NC, Elliott, AM and Sharp, L (2001) Rural and urban differences in stage at diagnosis of colorectal and lung cancers. *British Journal of Cancer*, 84: 910–14.

Care Quality Commission (CQC) (2009) *Voices into Action: Help make care better.* Available online at www.cqc.org.uk (accessed 15 December 2009).

Carpenter, M (1978) The new managerialism and professionalism in nursing, in Mackay, L, Soothill, K and Melia, K (1998) *Classic Texts in Health Care.* Oxford: Elsevier Health Science.

Carper, B (1978) Fundamental patterns of knowing in nursing. *Advances in Nursing Science*, 1: 13–23.

Cash, T, Gillen, B and Burns, D (1977) Sexism and 'beautyism' in personnel consultant decision making. *Journal of Applied Psychology*, 62: 301–10.

Centre for the Advancement of Interprofessional Learning (CAIPE) (1997) Interprofessional education: a definition. *CAIPE Bulletin*, 13: 19.

Centre for the Advancement of Interprofessional Learning (CAIPE) (2002) *Definition of Interprofessional Education and Learning.* London: CAIPE.

Chapman, A (no date) Johari window model. Available online at www.businessballs.com/johariwindowmodel.htm (accessed 8 February 2008).

Charatan, F (1997) US doctors and nurses clash over roles. *British Medical Journal*, 315: 899–904.

Chase, S (1995) The social context of critical care judgement. *Heart and Lung*, 24(2) (March/April): 154–62.

Chau, S, Humphreys, A, Wheeler, D, Cochrane, M, Skoda, S and Clement. S (2000) Nurse management of patients with minor illnesses in general practice: multicentre, randomised controlled trial. *British Medical Journal*, v(320): 1038–43.

Chesla, C (1996) Reconciling technologic and family care in critical care nursing. *Image Journal of Nursing Scholarship*, 28(3): 199–203.

CIPW (2007) *Creating an Interprofessional Workforce (CIPW).* London: NHS South West and Department of Health.

Clark, D (2008) 'Growing a team' Big Dog: Performance, learning, leadership and knowledge. Available online at www.nwlink.com/~donclark/leader/leadtem.html (accessed 13 February 2008).

Clark, M and Mills, J (1979) Interpersonal attraction in exchange and communal relationships. *Journal of Personality and Social Psychology*, 37: 12–24.

Clemow, R and Parker, M (2006) Webcast on authenticity and IPE for the Faculty of Health and Social Work, University of Plymouth. Available online at www.plymouth.ac.uk/pages/view.asp?page=4832 (accessed 10 March 2008).

Climate Change Act (2008) Available online at www.opsi.gov.uk/acts/acts2008/ukpga_20080027_en_1 (accessed 15 December 2009).

Cohen, H (1981) cited in Adams, K, Hean, S, Sturgis, P and Macleod, J (2006) Investigating the factors influencing professional identity of first year health and social care students. *Learning in Health and Social Care*, 5(2): 55–68.

Collings, K and Goodman, B (2003) The influence of multidisciplinary faculty on inter-professional learning. *Journal of Interprofessional Care*, 17(3) (August): 305.

Collins, N and Miller, L (1994) Self-disclosure and liking: a meta-analytic review. *Psychological Bulletin*, 116(3): 457–75.

Colyer, HM (2004) The construction and development of health professions: where will it end? *Journal of Advanced Nursing*, 48(4): 406–12.

Commission for Patient and Public Involvement in Health (CPPIH) (2007) Available online at www.cppih.org (accessed 8 February 2008).

Compact Oxford English Dictionary (COED) (2005) Third edition. Oxford: Oxford University Press.

Cooke, S, Wakefield, A, Chew- Graham, C and Boggis, C (2003) Collaborative training in breaking bad news to patients. *Journal of Interprofessional Care*, 17(3) (August): 307–8.

Coombs, M (2003) Power and conflict in intensive care, clinical decision making. *Intensive and Critical Care Nursing*, 19(3): 125–35.

Coombs, M and Ersser, S (2004) Medical hegemony in decision making: a barrier to working in intensive care? *Journal of Advanced Nursing*, 46(3) (May): 245–52.

Cooper, S, Carroll, J and Jenkin, A (2007) Collaborative practices in unscheduled emergency care: role and impact of the emergency care practitioner: qualitative and summative findings. *Emergency Medicine Journal*, 24(9) (September): 625–9.

Costello, A, Abbas, M and Allen, A et al. (2009) Managing the effects of climate change. *The Lancet*, 373: 1693–1733. Available online at www.thelancet.com/climate-change (accessed 15 December 2009).

Craig, P and Smith, L (1998) Health visiting and public health: back to our roots or a new branch? *Health and Social Care in the Community*, 6(3): 172–80.

Curley, C, McEachern, J and Speroff, T (1998) A firm trial of interdisciplinary rounds on the inpatient medical wards. *Medical Care*, 36 (suppl): AS4–12, in Zwarenstein, M and Reeves, S (2000) What's so great about collaboration? We need more evidence and less rhetoric, *British Medical Journal*, 320: 1022–3. Available at http://bmj.bmj journals.com/cgi/content/full/320/7241/1022 (accessed 12 February 2008).

Curtis, M (2004) Speak up about life and death issues. *Nursing Standard*, 18(52): 6.

D'Amour, D, Ferrada-Videla, M, San Martin Rodriguez, L and Beaulieu, M (2005) The conceptual basis for inter-professional collaboration: core concepts and theoretical frameworks. *Journal of Interprofessional Care*, Supplement 1: 116–31.

Darbyshire, P (1986) When the face doesn't fit. *Nursing Times*, 2 (April): 40–2.

Davenport, T and Prusak L (1998) *How Organizations Manage What They Know*. Boston, MA: Harvard Business School Press.

Davies, C (1995) *Gender and the Professional Predicament in Nursing*. Philadelphia, PA: Open University Press.

Davies, C (2000) Getting health professionals to work together. *British Medical Journal*, 320: 1021–2.

Day, J (2006) *Interprofessional Working*, Expanding Nursing and Health Care series (ed. L Wigens). Cheltenham: Nelson Thornes.

Dean, J (2008a) The halo effect: when your own mind is a mystery. PsyBlog. Available online at www.spring.org.uk/2007/10/halo-effect-when-your-own-mind-is.php (accessed 8 February 2008).

Dean, J (2008b) Getting closer: the art of self disclosure. PsyBlog. Available online at www.spring.org.uk/2007/02/getting-closer-art-of-self-disclosure.php (accessed 8 February 2008).

de Carlo, K (2007) Ogres and angels in the madhouse: mental health nursing identities in film. *International Journal of Mental Health Nursing*, 16(5) (October): 338–48.

D'Eon, MD (2005) A blueprint for interprofessional learning. *Journal of Interprofessional Care*, 19(S1): 49–59.

Department for Children, Schools and Families (DCSF) (2003) *Every Child Matters*. Available online at www.dcsf.gov.uk (accessed 15 December 2009).

Department for Children, Schools and Families (DCSF) (2004) *Every Child Matters: The next steps*. Available online at www.dcsf.gov.uk (accessed 15 December 2009).

Department for Education and Skills (DfES) (2004) *Every Child Matters: Change for children*. London: DfES.

Department of Health (DH) (1989a) *Caring for People: Community Care in the Next Decade and Beyond*. London: HMSO.

Department of Health (DH) (1989b) *Working for Patients*. London: HMSO.

Department of Health (DH) (1994) *Working in Partnership: A collaborative approach to care*, Report of the Mental Health Nursing Review Team. London: HMSO.

Department of Health (DH) (1996a) *The National Health Service: A service with ambitions*. London: HMSO.

Department of Health (DH) (1996b) *Primary Care: Delivering the Future*. London. HMSO.
Department of Health (DH) (1997) *The New NHS – Modern, Dependable*. London: HMSO.
Department of Health (DH) (1998) *A First Class Service: Quality in the new NHS*. London: HMSO.
Department of Health (DH) (1998a) *Modernising Mental Health Services: Safe, sound and supportive*. London: HMSO.
Department of Health (DH) (1998b) *Our Healthier Nation: A contract for health*, A Consultation Paper. London: HMSO.
Department of Health (DH) (1998c) *A First Class service: Quality in the new NHS*. London: HMSO.
Department of Health (DH) (1999) *Making a Difference. Strengthening the contribution of nurses, midwives and health visitors to health and health care*. London: HMSO.
Department of Health (DH) (2000a) *The NHS Plan: A plan for investment, a plan for reform*. London: HMSO.
Department of Health (DH) (2000b) *A Health Service of All the Talents: Developing the NHS Workforce*. London: HMSO.
Department of Health (DH) (2001) *National Service Frameworks for Older People*. London: HMSO.
Department of Health (DH) (2004) *The NHS Improvement Plan: Putting people at the heart of public services*. London: HMSO.
Department of Health (DH) (2005) *Working Time Directive Pilots Programme*, Final Report. London: NM Agency.
Department of Health (DH) (2006) *Our Health, Our Care, Our Say: A new direction for community services*. Available online at www.dh.gov.uk (accessed 8 February 2008).
Department of Health (DH) (2007a) *Local Involvement Networks Explained*. Available online at www.dh.gov.uk (accessed 8 February 2008).
Department of Health (DH) (2007b) *Our NHS, Our Future*, nationwide consultative event key findings, 18 September. Available online at www.ournhs.nhs.uk/fromtypepad/formatted_olr.pdf (accessed 8 February 2008).
Department of Health (DH) (2007c) *Review of NHS Service Improvement*, GNN, 28 February 2007. Available online at www.dh.gov.uk (accessed 8 February 2008).
Department of Health (DH) (2008a) *Our NHS: Next stage review – Leading local change*. London: Department of Health.
Department of Health (DH) (2008b) *High Quality Care for All: NHS next stage review, final report*. London: Department of Health.
Department of Health (DH) (2008c) *A High Quality Workforce: NHS next stage review*. London: Department of Health.
Department of Health (DH) (2008d) *Health Effects of Climate Change in the UK: An update of the Department of Health report 2001/2002*. Available online at www.dh.gov.uk (accessed 25 March 2009).
Department of Health (DH) (2008e) *The Health Impact of Climate Change: Promoting sustainable communities: Guidance document*, April. Available online at www.dh.gov.uk (accessed 25 March 2009).
Department of Health (DH) (2008f) *Taking the Long Term View: The Department of Health's strategy for delivering sustainable development 2008/2011*. Available online at www.dh.gov.uk (accessed 25 March 2009).
Department of Health (DH) (2009a) *The Engagement Cycle: A new way of thinking about patient and public engagement (PPE) in world-class commissioning*. Available online at www.dh.gov.uk (accessed 15 December 2009).
Department of Health (DH) (2009b) *Understanding What Matters: A guide to using patient feedback to transform care*. Available online at www.dh.gov.uk (accessed 15 December 2009).
Department of Health (DH) (2009c) *Putting Patients at the Heart of Care*. Available online at www.dh.gov.uk (accessed 15 December 2009).

Department of Health (DH) (2009d) *Helping the NHS Put Patients at the Heart of Care.* Available online at www.dh.gov.uk (accessed 15 December 2009).

Department of Health (DH) (2009e) *Real Accountability: Guidance on the NHS duty to involve.* Available online at www.dh.gov.uk (accessed 15 December 2009).

Department of Health (DH) (2009f) *Safeguarding Adults: Report on the consultation on the review of 'No Secrets'.* London: Department of Health.

Department of Health and Social Services (DHSS) (1974) *Report of the Committee of Inquiry into the Care and Supervision Provided in Relation to Maria Colwell.* London: DHSS.

Devendra, S and Randall, P (2007) Beauty is in the eye of the plastic surgeon: waist–hip ratio and women's attractiveness. *Personality and Individual Differences*, 43(2): 329–40.

Diamond, P (2007) The brave new world of government reform. *The Guardian*, 30 May 2007. Available online at http://society.guardian.co.uk/publicmanager/story/0,,2090 538,00.html (accessed 8 February 2008).

Dickenson, A (2006) Implementing the single assessment process: opportunities and challenges. *Journal of Interprofessional Care*, 20(4): 365–79.

Dion, K, Berscheid, E and Webster, E (1972) What is beautiful is good. *Journal of Personality and Social Psychology*, 24: 285–90.

Douglas, C (2000) Nursing matters. *British Medical Journal*, 320: 1085.

Ebbs, N and Timmons, S (2007) Interprofessional working in the RAF Critical Care Air Support Team (CCAST). *Intensive and Critical Care Nursing*. Available online at doi:10.1016/j.iccn.2007.06.003.

Economic and Social Research Council (ESRC) (2005) Telemedicine revolution is 'disappearing' from the NHS, ESRC, 30 June 2007. Available online at www.esrc societytoday.ac.uk (accessed 8 February 2008).

Elliott, L and Atkinson, D (2007) *Fantasy Island: Waking up to the incredible economic, political and social illusions of the Blair legacy.* London: Constable.

Elston, S and Holloway, I (2001) The impact of recent primary care reforms in the UK on interprofessional working in primary care centres. *Journal of Interprofessional Care*, 15(1): 19–27.

Etzioni, A (1969) *The Semi Professions and their Organisation.* New York: The Free Press.

European Commission (2000) *New Community Health Strategy: Communication from the Commission to the Council, the European Parliament, the Economic and Social Committee and the Committee of the Regions on the health strategy of the European Community*, COM/2000/0285 final. Available online at http://europa. eu/scadplus/leg/en/cha/c11563.htm (accessed 8 February 2008).

Evans, J (2002) Cautious caregivers: gender stereotypes and the sexualization of men nurses' touch. *Journal of Advanced Nursing*, 40(4) (November): 441–8.

Fahrenwald, N, Bassett, S, Tschetter, L, Carson, P, White, L and Winterboer, V (2005) Teaching core nursing values. *Journal of Professional Nursing*, 21(1) (January/ February): 46–51.

Ferns, T and Chojnacka, I (2005) Angels and swingers, matrons and sinners: nursing stereotypes. *British Journal of Nursing*, 14(1): 1028–32.

Festinger, L (1957) *A Theory of Cognitive Dissonance.* Stanford, CA: Stanford University Press. Also available online at http://home.sprynet.com/~gkearsley.

Finch, J (2000) Interprofessional education and teamworking: a view from the education providers. *British Medical Journal*, 321: 1138–40.

Finke, S (2004) *Social Beings: A core motives approach to social psychology.* New York: John Wiley.

Firth-Cozens, J (1990) Sources of stress in women junior house officers. *British Medical Journal*, 301: 89–91.

Fisak, B, Tantleff-Dunn, S and Peterson, R (2007) Personality information: does it influence attractiveness ratings of various body sizes? *BodyImage*, 4(2) (June): 213–17.

Fisher, S, Hunter, T and MacRosson, W (2001) A validation study of Belbin's team roles. *European Journal of Work and Organizational Psychology*, 10(2): 121–44.

Ford, M and Walsh, P (1990) *Nursing Rituals Research and Rational Action*. London: Butterworth Heinemann.

Freeth, D, Hammick, M, Koppel, I, Reeves, S and Barr, H. (2002) *A Critical Review of Evaluations of Interprofessional Education*, commissioned by LTSN, HS&P. London: CAIPE.

Freeth, D, Hammick, M, Reeves, S, Koppel, I and Barr, H (2005) *Effective Interprofessional Education: Development, delivery and evaluation*. Oxford: Blackwell.

Friedson, E (1970) *Profession of Medicine*. Chicago, IL: University of Chicago Press.

Furnham, A, Steele, H and Pendleton, D (1993) A psychometric assessment of the Belbin Team-Role Self-Perception Inventory. *Journal of Occupational and Organizational Psychology*, 66(3): 245–57.

Gamarnikow, E. (1978) Sexual division of labour: the case of nursing, in Kuhn, A and Wolpe, AM (eds) *Feminism and Materialism: Women and modes of production*. London: Routledge and Kegan Paul.

Garfinkel, H (1967) *Studies in Ethnomethodology*. Malden, MA: Blackwell.

Gilbert, J (2005) Interprofessional learning and higher education structural barriers. *Journal of Interprofessional Care*, 19(s1): 87–106.

Gilbert, J, Camp, R, Cole, C, Bruce, C, Fielding, D and Stanton, S (2000) Preparing students for interprofessional teamwork in health care. *Journal of Interprofessional Care*, 14(3): 223–35.

Gill, M, Goodlee, F, Horton, R and Stott, R (2007) Doctors and climate change. *British Medical Journal*, 335: 1104–5.

Glenn, T, Rhea, J and Wheeless, L (1997) Interpersonal communication satisfaction and biologic sex: nurse-physician relationships. *Communication Research Reports* 14(1): 24–32.

Goffman, E (1959) *The Presentation of Self in Everyday Life*. New York: Doubleday.

Goldenberg, D and Iwasiw, C (1993) Professional socialisation of nursing students as an outcome of a senior clinical preceptorship. *Nurse Education Today* 13(1): 3–15.

Goleman, D (1995) *Emotional Intelligence: Why it can matter more than IQ*. London: Bloomsbury.

Goodman, B (2002) Ms B and legal competence: examining the role of nurses in difficult ethico-legal decision making. *Nursing in Critical Care*, 8(2) (March/April): 78–83.

Goodman, B (2004) Ms B and legal competence: interprofessional collaboration and nurse autonomy. *Nursing in Critical Care*, 9(6): 271–6.

Goodman, B (2006) Head and hands. *Nursing Standard*, 20(19): 69.

Goodman, B and Richardson, J (2010) In press.

Goodman, B and Strange, F (1997) Ethnomethodology, in Smith, P (ed.) *Research Mindedness for Practice: An interactive approach for nursing and health*. Edinburgh: Churchill Livingstone.

Griffiths, K (2000) The role of categorisation in perception. Available online at www.aber.ac.uk/media/Students/klg9901.html (accessed 8 February 2008).

Griffiths, J (2007) *Proceedings of the Faculty of Public Health Conference*, 27 June. Available online at www.publichealthconferences.org.uk (accessed 25 March 2009).

Gross, R and Kinnison, N (2007) *Psychology for Nurses and Allied Health Professionals*. London: Hodder Arnold.

Guardian, The (2007) A matter of choice. Available online at www.guardian.co.uk/society/2007/may/30/publicservices.politics (accessed 12 February 2008).

Hall, B (2004) Fight your corner. *Nursing Standard*, 18(35): 18–19.

Hammick, M, Freeth, D, Koppel, I, Reeves, S and Barr, H (2007) A best evidence systematic review of interprofessional education. *Medical Teacher*, 29: 735–51.

Hansen, J, Mik Sato, P, Kharencha, G, Russell, D, Lea, W and Siddall, M (2007) Climate change and trace gases. *Philosophical Transactions of the Royal Society A*, 365: 1925–54.

Healthcare Commission (2003) *Harold Shipman's Clinical Practice 1974–1998: A clinical audit commissioned by the Chief Medical Officer*. London: Healthcare Commission.

Healthcare Commission (2006) *Investigation into 10 Maternal Deaths at, or following, Delivery at Northwick Park Hospital, North West London Hospitals NHS Trust, between April 2002 and April 2005*. London: Healthcare Commission.

Heenan, A (1991) cited in Sweet, S and Norman, I (1995) The nurse–doctor relationship: a selective literature review. *Journal of Advanced Nursing*, 22: 165–70.

Henderson, A, van Eps, M and Pearson, K (2007) 'Caring for' behaviours that indicate to patients that nurses 'care about' them. *Journal of Advanced Nursing*, 60(2) (October): 146–53.

Hochschild, A (2003) *The Managed Heart: Commercialization of human feeling*, 2nd edition. Berkeley, CA: University of Californa Press.

Hornby, S and Atkins, J (2000) *Collaborative Care: Interprofessional, interagency and interpersonal*. Oxford: Blackwell.

Horsburgh, M and Perkins, R (2006) The professional substructures of students entering medicine, nursing and pharmacy programmes. *Journal of Interprofessional Care*, 20(4): 425–31.

Houston, A and Cowley, S (2002) An empowerment approach to health needs assessment in health visiting practice. *Journal of Clinical Nursing*, 11: 640–50.

Hovland, C, Janis, I and Kelley, H (1953) *Communication and Persuasion*. New Haven, CT: Yale University Press. Also available online at http://home.sprynet.com/~gkearsley.

Howarth, M, Holland, K and Grant, MJ (2006) Educational needs for integrated care: a literature review, in *Integrated Literature Reviews and Meta-analysis: The Authors' Journal Compilation*. Oxford: Blackwell, pp144–56.

Hughes, D (1988) When nurses know best: some aspects of nurse–doctor interaction in a casualty department. *Sociology of Health and Illness*, 10: 1–22.

Hussein, E (2007) *The Islamist*. London: Penguin.

Intergovernmental Panel on Climate Change (IPCC) (2007) *Climate Change 2007: The Physical Science Basis: Summary for policy makers*. Geneva: IPCC Secretariat. Available online at www.ippc.ch (accessed 15 January 2009).

James, O (2007) *Affluenza*. London: Vermilion.

Jitapunkul, S, Nuchprayoon, C, Aksaranugraha, S, Chalwanichsiri, D, Leenawat, B and Kotepong, W (1995) A controlled clinical trial of multidisciplinary team approach in the general medical wards of Chulalongkorn Hospital. *Journal of the Medical Association Thailand*, 78: 618–23 [Medline] in Zwarenstein, M and Reeves, S (2000) What's so great about collaboration? We need more evidence and less rhetoric. *British Medical Journal*, 320: 1022–3. Available online at http://bmj.bmjjournals. com/cgi/content/full/320/7241/1022 (accessed 10 June 2005)

Jones, A (2003) Changes in practice at the nurse-doctor interface: using focus groups to explore the perceptions of first level nurses working in an acute care setting. *Journal of Clinical Nursing* 12(1) (January): 124–31.

Jones, A (2006) Multidisciplinary team working: collaboration and conflict. *International Journal of Mental Health Nursing*, 15(1) (March): 19–28.

Kahneman, D, Slovic, P and Tversky, A (1982) cited in Buckingham, C (2000) Classifying clinical decision making: a unifying approach. *Journal of Advanced Nursing*, 32(4) (October): 981–9.

Kearsley, G (2007) *Cognitive Dissonance (L Festinger) Explorations in Learning & Instruction: The theory into practice database*. Available online at http://tip. psychology.org (accessed 8 February 2008).

Kelley, H (1950) The warm-cold variable in first impressions of people. *Journal of Personality*, 18: 431–9.

Kelso, P. (2001) The cool one who did not cry. *The Guardian*, 23 June. Available online at www.guardian.co.uk/bulger/article/0,,511450,00.html (accessed 8 February 2008).

Kennedy, I (2001) *The Inquiry into the Management of the Care of Children Receiving Complex Heart Surgery at the Bristol Royal Infirmary*. London: Department of Health.

Kinnersley, P, Anderson, E, Parry, K, Clement, J, Archard, L, Turton, P, Stainthorpe, A, Fraser, E, Butler, C and Rogers, C (2000) Randomised controlled trial of nurse practitioner versus general practitioner care for patients requesting 'same day' consultations in primary care. *British Medical Journal*, 320: 1043–8.

Kleffel, D (2004) Advocating the ecocentric paradigm in nursing. *Journal of Holistic Nursing*, 22(1): 6–10.

Kristainsen, L, Dahl, A, Asplund, K and Hellzen, O (2005) The impact of nurses' opinion of client behaviour and level of social functioning on the amount of time they spend with clients. *Journal of Psychiatric and Mental Health Nursing*, 12(6): 719–27.

Kruijver, I, Kerkstra, A, Bensing, J and van de Wiel, H (2001) Communication skills of nurses during interactions with simulated cancer patients. *Journal of Advanced Nursing*, 34(6): 772–9.

Ladyman, S (2004) Speech to Practice Learning Taskforce, Parliamentary Under Secretary of State for Community, 25 March. Available online at www.dh.gov.uk/en/News/Speeches/Speecheslist/DH_4078447 (accessed 27 May 2008).

Lagos, T (2009) *Global Citizenship: Towards a definition*. Available online at http://depts.washington.edu/gcp/pdf/globalcitizenship.pdf (accessed 15 December 2009).

Laming, Lord (2003) *The Victoria Climbié Inquiry: Report of an inquiry by Lord Laming*. London: Department of Health.

Langley, G, Nolan, K and Nolan, T (1992) *The Foundation of Improvement*. Silver Spring, MD: API Publishing.

Langley, G, Nolan, K, Norman, C and Provost, L (2000) *The Improvement Guide: A practical approach to enhancing organisational performance*. San Francisco, CA: Jossey Bass.

Langlois, JH, Kalakanis, L, Rubenstein, AJ, Larson, A and Hallam, M (2000) cited in Devendra, S and Randall, P (2007) Beauty is in the eye of the plastic surgeon: waist hip ratio (WHR) and women's attractiveness. *Personality and Individual Differences*, 43: 329–40.

Leathard, A (1994) *Going Inter-professional: Working together for health and welfare*. London: Routledge.

Leathard, A (ed.) (2003) *Inter-professional Collaboration: From policy to practice in health and social care*. Hove: Brunner Routledge.

Lennox, A and Anderson, E (2007) *The Leicester Model of Interprofessional Education: A practical guide for implementation in health and social care*. Newcastle: University of Newcastle, Higher Education Academy Subject Centre for Medicine, Dentistry and Veterinary Medicine.

Levy, B, Ashman, O and Dror, I (2000) To be or not to be: the effects of aging stereotypes on the will to live. *Omega*, 40(3): 409–20.

Lorenz, K (2005) Do pretty people earn more? Available online at www.cnn.com/2005/US/Careers/07/08/looks/ (accessed 8 February 2008).

Luchins, A (1957) Primacy–recency in impression formation, in Hovland, C (ed.) *The Order of Presentation in Persuasion*, New Haven, CT: Yale University Press.

Luke, H (2003) *Medical Education and Sociology of Medical Habitus: Its not about the stethoscope*. Dordrecht: Springer.

McCallin, A (2001) Interdisciplinary practice – a matter of teamwork: an integrated literature review. *Journal of Clinical Nursing*, 10(4): 419–28.

McCallin, A and Bamford, A (2007) Interdisciplinary teamwork: is the influence of emotional intelligence fully appreciated? *Journal of Nursing Management*, 15: 386–91.

McCann, K and McKenna, H (1993) An examination of touch between nurses and elderly patients in a continuing care setting in Northern Ireland. *Journal of Advanced Nursing*, 18(5): 838–46.

McGregor, D (2008) cited in Clark, D (2008) *'Growing a team' Big Dog: Performance, learning, leadership and knowledge.* Available online at www.nwlink.com/~donclark/leader/leadtem.html (accessed 13 February 2008).

MacIntosh, J and Dingwall, R (1978) cited in Speed, S and Luker, K (2006) Getting a visit: how district nurses and general practitioners 'organise' each other in primary care. *Sociology of Health and Illness,* 28(7): 883–902. Available online at doi: 10.1111/j.1467-9566.2006.00511.x.

Mackay, L (1993) cited in Sweet, S and Norman, I (1995) The nurse–doctor relationship: a selective literature review, *Journal of Advanced Nursing,* 22: 165–70.

Mackay, L (1995) The patient as pawn, in Soothill, K, Mackay, L and Webb, C (eds) *Interprofessional Relations in Health Care.* London: Arnold.

Mackintosh, C (2006) Caring: the socialisation of pre-registration student nurses: a longitudinal study. *International Journal of Nursing Studies,* 43(8): 953–62.

McLuhan, M (1994) *Understanding Media: The extensions of man.* Cambridge, MA: MIT Press.

McMichael, AJ and Powells, JW (1999) Human numbers, enjoyment, sustainability and health. *British Medical Journal,* 319: 1977–80.

McParland, J, Scott, PA and Arndt, M (2000) Autonomy and clinical practice 3: issues of patient consent. *British Journal of Nursing,* 9(10): 660–5.

McPherson, K, Headrick, L and Moss, F (2001) Working together, learning together: good quality care depends on it, but how can we achieve it? *Quality in Health Care,* 10 (supplement II): 46–53.

Manias, E and Street, A (2001) The interplay of knowledge and decision making between nurses and doctors in critical care. *International Journal of Nursing Studies,* 38(2): 129–40.

Manktelow, J (2003) www.mindtools.com.

Marconi, J (2001) *Reputation Marketing.* Menlo Park, CA. McGraw Hill.

Margerison, C and McCann, D (1985) *How to Lead a Winning Team.* Bradford: MCB University Press.

Marshall, M and Rathbone, J (2004) Early intervention for psychosis. Cochrane Database of Systematic Reviews, Issue 2, Art. No.: CD004718. Available online at www.cochrane.org/reviews/en/ab004718.html (accessed 8 February 2008).

Martin, G. (1998) Empowerment of dying patients: the strategies and barriers to patient autonomy. *Journal of Advanced Nursing,* 28(4) (October): 737–44.

Martin-Rodriguez, LS, Beaulieu, MD, D'Armour, D and Ferrada-Videla, M (2005) The determinants of successful collaboration: a review of theoretical and empirical studies. *Journal of Interprofessional Care,* s1: 132–47.

Mayor, S (2006) Health secretary pledges to continue NHS changes. *British Medical Journal,* 333: 617.

Melia, K (1984) Student nurses' construction of occupational socialisation. *Sociology of Health and Illness,* 6(2): 132–51.

Melia, K (1987) *Working and Learning: The occupational socialisation of nurses.* London: Tavistock.

Messerli-Rohrbach, V (2000) Personal values and medical preferences: postmaterialism, spirituality, and the use of complementary medicine. *Forsch Komplementarmed,* 7(4) (August): 183–9.

Mickan, S and Rodger, S (2005) Effective health care teams: a model of six characteristics developed from shared perceptions. *Journal of Interprofessional Care,* 19(4) (August): 358–70.

Miller, C (2004) *Producing Welfare: A modern agenda.* Basingstoke: Palgrave Macmillan.

Mitchell, P (1994) What's up doc? *Nursing Standard,* 8(32): 54–5.

Monkton Report, The (1948) in Day, J. (2006) *Interprofessional Working,* Expanding Nursing and Health Care series (ed. L Wigens). Cheltenham: Nelson Thornes.

Mrayyan, M (2004) Nurses' autonomy: influence of nurse managers' actions. *Nursing and Healthcare Management and Policy,* 45(3): 326.

Muldoon, O. (2003) Career choice in nursing students: gendered constructs as psychological barriers. *Journal of Advanced Nursing*, 43(1) (July): 93–100.

NHS Executive (1996) *Primary Care: The future*. London: NHSME.

NHS Institute for Innovation and Improvement. Available online at www.institute.nhs.uk/ (accessed 13 February 2008).

Nisbett, R and Ross, L (1980) cited in Gross, R and Kinnison, N (2007) *Psychology for Nurses and Allied Health Professionals*. London: Hodder Arnold.

Nisbett, R and Wilson, T (1977) The halo effect: evidence for unconscious alteration of judgments. *Journal of Personality and Social Psychology*, 35(4): 250–6.

Nursing and Midwifery Council (NMC) (2004) *The NMC Code of Professional Conduct: Standards for conduct, performance and ethics*. London: NMC. Also available online at www.nmc-uk.org.

Nursing and Midwifery Council (NMC) (2004a) *Standards of Proficiency for Pre-registration Nursing Education*. London: NMC.

Nursing and Midwifery Council (NMC) (2006) *Standards to Support Learning and Assessment in Practice*. London: NMC. Available online at www.nmc-uk.org/ (accessed 13 February 2008).

Nursing and Midwifery Council (NMC) (2007) Essential skills clusters (ESCs) for pre-registration nursing programmes. Annexe 2 to NMC circular 07/2007. Available online at www.nmc-uk.org (accessed 27 May 2008).

Nursing and Midwifery Council (NMC) (2008) *The Code: Standards for conduct, performance and ethics*. London: NMC. Also available online at www.nmc-uk.org.

Nursing and Midwifery Council (NMC) (2010) *Draft Standards for Pre-registration Nursing Education*. London: NMC. Available online at www.nmc-uk.org/ (accessed 15 February 2010).

Oakley, A. (1995) Doctor knows best, in Davey, B, Gray, A and Seale, C (eds) *Health and Disease: A reader*, 2nd edition. Buckingham: Open University Press.

O'Dowd, A (2007) Carruthers report calls for doctors to be more involved in NHS change. *British Medical Journal* 334: 499.

Orem, DE (1985) *Nursing: Concepts of practice*. Menlo Park, CA: McGraw Hill.

Orr, D (1994) *Earth in Mind: On education, environment and the human project*. Washington, DC: Island Press.

Øvretveit, J, Mathias, P and Thompson, T (1997) *Interprofessional Working for Health and Social Care*. London: Macmillan.

Oxtoby, K (2003) What's your stereotype? *Nursing Times*, 99(41): 34–6.

Parcell, G, Gibbs, T and Bligh, J (1998) The visual techniques to enhance interprofessional learning. *Postgraduate Medical Journal*, 74(873): 387–90.

Peplau, HE (1988) *Interpersonal Relations in Nursing: A conceptual frame of reference for psychodynamic nursing*. Basingstoke: Macmillan Education.

Pietroni, P (1992) Towards reflective practice: the language of health and social care. *Journal of Interprofessional Care*, 6: 7–16.

Podcasts. Available online at www.health.heacademy.ac.uk/ipe.

Porter, S (1991) cited in Sweet, S and Norman, I (1995) The nurse–doctor relationship: a selective literature review. *Journal of Advanced Nursing*, 22: 165–70.

Pringle, R (1996) Nursing a grievance: women doctors and nurses. *Journal of Gender Studies*, 5(2): 157–68.

Pringle, R (1998) *Sex and Medicine: Gender, power and authority in the medical profession*. Cambridge: Cambridge University Press.

Quality Assurance Agency (QAA) (2006) *Statement of Common Purpose for Subject Benchmarks for Health and Social Care*. Gloucester: QAA.

Radcliffe, M (2000) Doctors and nurses: new game same result. *British Medical Journal*, 320: 1085.

Rawson, D (1994) Models of interprofessional work: likely theories and possibilities, in Day, J (2006) *Interprofessional Working*, Expanding Nursing and Health Care series (ed. L Wigens). Cheltenham: Nelson Thornes.

Rayner, F (2003) Are nurses ready to take over junior doctors' roles? *Nursing Times*, 99: 10–11.

Robbins, H and Finlay, M (2000) *The New Why Teams Don't Work: What goes wrong and how to make it right*. San Francisco, CA: Berrett-Koehler.

Roper, N, Logan, WW and Tierney, A (1980) *The Elements of Nursing*. Edinburgh: Churchill Livingstone.

Rosenstein, A (2002) Nurse–physician relationships: impact on nurse satisfaction and retention. *American Journal of Nursing*, 102(6): 26–34.

Rothstein, W and Hannum, S (2007) Profession and gender relationships between advanced nurses and physicians. *Journal of Professional Nursing*, 23(4): 235–40.

Roy, C (1980) Conceptual Models for Nursing Practice. [[PLACE?]]: Appelton Century.

Royal College of Nursing (RCN) (2006) *Principles: A framework for evaluating health and social care policy*. London: RCN.

Salvage, J and Smith, R (2000) Doctors and nurses: doing it differently. *British Medical Journal*, 320: 1019–20.

Sawatzky, J (1996) Stress in critical care nurses: actual and perceived. *Heart Lung*, 25: 409–17.

Schumacher, E (1973, 2nd edn 1993) *Small is Beautiful*, London: Vintage.

Scottish Telemedicine Initiative (2000) Available online at www.telemedicine.scot. nhs.uk/ (accessed 8 February 2008).

Seebohm Report, The (1968) cited in Day, J. (2006) *Interprofessional Working*, Expanding Nursing and Health Care series (ed. L Wigens). Cheltenham: Nelson Thornes.

Senge, PM (1990) *The Fifth Discipline: The art and practice of the learning organization*. London: Random House. Available online at www.infed.org/thinkers/senge.htm#_ The_learning_organization) (accessed 13 February 2008).

Shipman Inquiry, The (2005) Systems failures and tasks for phase two, Section 14.16. Available online at www.the-shipman-inquiry.org.uk/home.asp (accessed 8 February 2008).

Sinclair, F (2009) *What is Sustainability?* Available online at http://ecohearth.com/eco-news/eco-op-ed/300-what-is-sustainability.html (accessed 25 March 2009).

Sitzia, J, Cotterell, P and Richardson, A (2006) Interprofessional collaboration with service users in the development of cancer services: the cancer partnership project. *Journal of Interprofessional Care*, 20(1) (January): 60–74.

Skjorshammer, M (2001) Co-operation and conflict in a hospital: inter-professional differences in perception and management of conflicts. *Journal of Interprofessional Care*, 15(1): 7–18

Sleutel, M (2000) Intrapartum nursing care: a case study of supportive interventions and ethical conflicts. *Birth*, 27(1): 38–45. Available online at http://angelo.edu/faculty/ msleutel/pdf/birth.pdf (accessed 10 June 2005).

Smith, P. (1992) *The Emotional Labour of Nursing: Its impact on interpersonal relations, management and the educational environment in nursing*. Basingstoke: Macmillan.

Snelgrove, S and Hughes, D (2000) Inter-professional relations between doctors and nurses: perspectives from South Wales. *Journal of Advanced Nursing*, 31(3): 661–7.

Snyder, M (1974) Self-monitoring of expressive behaviour. *Journal of Personality and Social Psychology*, 30: 526–37. Available online at http://pubpages.unh.edu/~ckb/ SELFMON2.html (accessed 8 February 2008).

Sorlie, V, Torjuul, K, Ross, A and Kihlgren, M (2006) Satisfied patients are also vulnerable patients: narratives from an acute care ward. *Journal of Clinical Nursing* 15(10): 1240–6.

Speed, S and Luker, K (2006) Getting a visit: how district nurses and general practitioners 'organise' each other in primary care. *Sociology of Health and Illness*, 28(7): 883–902. Available online at doi: 10.1111/j.1467–9566.2006.00511.x.

Spurgeon, D (1996) Canadian doctors challenge nurses' expanded role. *British Medical Journal*, 313: 1033.

Stacey, M and Reid, M (eds) *Health and the Division of Labour*. London: Croomfield.

Stanley, J (1998) Mixed messages. *Nursing Times*, 94(9) (December): 58–9.

Stein, L (1967) The doctor–nurse game. *Archive of General Psychiatry*, 16: 699–703.

Stein, L, Watts, D and Howell, T (1990) The doctor–nurse game revisited. *New England Journal of Medicine*, 322: 546–9 in Zelek, B and Phillips, S (2003) Gender and power: nurses and doctors in Canada. *International Journal for Equity in Health*, 2(1). Available online at www.equityhealthj.com/content/2/1/1 (accessed 10 June 2005).

Stern, H, Stroh, S, Fiser, D and Cromwell, S (1991) Communication, decision making and perception of nursing roles in a paediatric intensive care unit. *Critical Care Nurses Quarterly*, 14(3): 56–68.

Stockwell, F (1972) *The Unpopular Patient*. London: Royal College of Nursing.

Sum, C, Humphreys, A, Wheeler, D, Cochrane, M, Skoda, S and Clement, S (2000) Nurse management of patients with minor illnesses in general practice: multicentre, randomised controlled trial. *British Medical Journal*, 320: 1038–43.

Sundin-Huard, D (2001) Subject positions theory: its application to understanding collaboration (and confrontation) in critical care. *Journal of Advanced Nursing*, 34(3): 376–82.

Sustainable Development Commission (2009) *About Sustainable Development*. Available online at www.sd-commission.org.uk (accessed 15 December 2009).

Svensonn, R (1996) The interplay between doctors and nurses: a negotiated order perspective. *Sociology of Health and Illness*, 18: 370–98.

Sweet, S and Norman, I (1995) The nurse–doctor relationship: a selective literature review. *Journal of Advanced Nursing*, 22: 165–70.

Tabak, N and Orit, K (2007) Relationship between how nurses resolve their conflicts with doctors, their stress and satisfaction. *Journal of Nursing Management*, 15(3) (April).

Tajfel, H (1974) Social identity and intergroup behaviour. *Social Science Information*, 13: 65–93.

Tannen, D (1994) *Talking from 9 to 5: How women's and men's conversational styles affect who gets heard, who gets credit, and what gets done at work*. New York: William Morrow and Company, pp123–4, in Zelek, B and Phillips, S (2003) Gender and power: nurses and doctors in Canada. *International Journal for Equity in Health*, 2(1). Available online at www.equityhealthj.com/content/2/1/1 (accessed 10 June 2005).

Taylor, C (1992) *The Ethics of Authenticity*. Cambridge, MA: Harvard University Press.

Taylor, M (2009) *A New Politics: Citizens not consumers*. Available online at www.guardian.co.uk/commentisfree/2009/jun/a-new-politics-constitutional-reform2 (accessed 15 December 2009).

Thompson, C (2003) Clinical experience as evidence in evidence-based practice. *Journal of Advanced Nursing*, 43(3): 230–7.

Thompson, DR and Stewart, S (2007) Handmaiden or right-hand man: is the relationship between doctors and nurses still therapeutic? *International Journal of Cardiology*, 118(2): 139–40.

Tietje, L and Cresap, S (2005) Is lookism unjust? The ethics of aesthetics and public policy implications. *Journal of Libertarian Studies* 19(2): 31–50.

Tucker, R (2004) *Another Gospel: Cults, alternative religions, and the New Age movement*. Grand Rapids, MI: Zondervan.

Tuckman, BW (1965) Developmental sequence in small groups. *Psychological Bulletin*, 63: 384–99.

Tuckman, BW and Jensen, MA (1977) Stages of small group development revisited. *Group and Organisational Studies*, 2: 419–27.

Tyke, J (2004) The weaker sex? *Practice Nurse*, 27(8) (April): 74.

Universities UK (2003) *Partners in Care: Universities and the NHS*. London: Universities UK.

Vyt, A (2009) *Exploring Quality Assurance for Interprofessional Education in Health and Social Care*. London: Garant.

Walby, S, Greenwell, J, Mackay, L and Soothill, K (1994) *Medicine and Nursing: Professions in a changing health service*, London: Sage.

Walsh, C, Gordon, F, Marshall, M, Wilson, F and Hunt, T (2005) Interprofessional capability: a framework for interprofessional education. *Nurse Education in Practice*, 5(4): 230–7.

Watson, T (2003) *Sociology, Work and Industry*, 4th edition. London: Routledge.

Wellins, R, William, B and Wilson, J (1991) *Empowered Teams: Creating self-directed work groups that improve quality, productivity, and participation*. San Francisco, CA: Jossey-Bass.

World Health Organization (WHO) (1978) International Conference on Primary Health Care. Declaration of Alma-Ata. Available online at www.who.int (accessed 5 January 2008).

Willard, B (1993) *Team Resources: Annual leadership development handout*. IBM Canada Leadership Development, rgwilla@ibm.net. Available online at www.strategy2reality.com (accessed 13 February 2008).

Wiman, E and Wikblad, K (2004) Caring and uncaring encounters in nursing in an emergency department. *Journal of Clinical Nursing*, 13(4): 422–9.

Witz, A (1992) *Professions and Patriarchy*. London: Routledge.

Woodham Smith, C (1952) cited in Thompson, D and Stewart, S (2007) Handmaiden or right-hand man: is the relationship between doctors and nurses still therapeutic? *International Journal of Cardiology*, 118(2)(31): 139–40.

World Health Organization (WHO) (2006) *The World Health Report: Working together for health*. Geneva: World Health Organization.

World Health Organization (WHO) (2009) *WHO Framework for Action on Interprofessional Education & Collaborative Practice*. Geneva: WHO. Available online at www2.rgu.ac.uk/ipe/WHO_report_Interprofessional%20Ed%20Sep2509.pdf (accessed 8 January 2010).

Wright, S (2004) Say goodbye to core values. *Nursing Standard*, 18(34): 22–3.

Xyrichis, A and Ream, E (2008) Teamwork: a concept analysis. *Journal of Advanced Nursing*, 61(2): 231–41.

Yan, J, Gilbert, JH and Hoffman, SJ (2007) WHO study group on interprofessional education and collaborative practice. *Journal of Interprofessional Care*, 21(6): 588–9.

Zelek, B and Phillips, S (2003) Gender and power: nurses and doctors in Canada. *International Journal for Equity in Health*, 2(1). Available online at www.equityhealthj.com/content/2/1/1 (accessed 10 June 2005).

Zwarenstein, M and Reeves, S (2000) What's so great about collaboration? We need more evidence and less rhetoric. *British Medical Journal*, 320: 1022–3. Available online at http://bmj.bmjjournals.com/cgi/content/full/320/7241/1022 (accessed 10 June 2005).

Zwarenstein, M and Bryant, W. (2000) Interventions to improve collaboration between nurses and doctors, in Bero, L, Grilli, R, Grimshaw, J, Oxman, A and Zwarenstein, M (eds) Cochrane Collaboration on effective professional practice module of the Cochrane database of systematic reviews, in Cochrane Collaboration, *Cochrane Library*, Issue 2. Oxford: Update Software.

Zwarenstein, S, Reeves, S, Barr, H, Hammick, M, Koppel, I and Atkins, J (2000). *Interprofessional Education: Effects on professional practice and health*. Oxford: The Cochrane Library.

Index

In the following index, material in Activity boxes has often been included.